Anti-Inflammatory Diet for Beginners

Planted Based and Hight Protein Nutrition Guide (with 100+ Delicious Recipes)

I0223247

Nancy Welch

Introduction

Have you been feeling sluggish and sore just getting out of bed in the morning? Sick of feeling tired and achy everyday? Looking for a sustainable way to lose weight, eat healthy, and gain back your lost energy?

Well then, congratulations on taking your first step to healthy living by purchasing*The Anti-Inflammatory Diet for Beginnersbook,* and thank you for doing so!

The following chapters will discuss how to improve your daily life, heal your immune system, lose weight, and even prevent degenerative diseases. Inflammation can throw you into a cycle that is difficult to get out of, causing pain in your muscles and joints, leaving you less active. Living a more sedentary lifestyle will cause weight gain, which will then put more pressure on your joints and cause more inflammation. But, you can control the inflammation by just making a few adjustments to what and how you eat.

It takes only takes 3 weeks to make anything a habit, start today and build a strong, healthy future.Included is a 3-week meal plan with breakfast, lunch, dinner, smoothies, and even dessert recipes. By just changing your way of eating, you can reduce the inflammation that causes fatigue, joint pain, slowed cognitive function, and many autoimmune diseases. You will find you no longer need pain medication daily,and you don't have to starve yourself to get there!

There are many books available to you on this subject, again, thank you for selecting this one! A great deal of effort was made to ensure this book was an easy read while still full of as much useful information as possible; please enjoy!

Chapter 1: What is Inflammation?

Inflammation is part of the body's reaction to an injury or infection. It is a physiological response that alerts your immune system that it needs to repair damaged cells or fight off viruses and bacteria. Without inflammation signaling your immune system to go to work, infected wounds, and viruses would be deadly.

Unfortunately, it is not a perfect system. Sometimes the inflammation will flare up in parts of the body where it is not needed. This can lead to chronic inflammation, which has been linked to stroke, heart disease, and autoimmune disorders.

There are two different types of inflammation, acute and chronic. Acute inflammation is what occurs after being injured, such as a scratch or cut, twisted ankle, or even a sore throat. This would trigger the immune system to react to the injured area only. The inflammation would only last as long as needed to repair the damage. It would cause the red blood vessels to dilate and increase blood flow. White blood cells would increase in the area needed and help to heal the body. You may see the signs of acute inflammation such as redness, swelling, pain, and the area may feel warm to the touch or cause a fever.

When there is acute inflammation, the damaged tissue releases a chemical called cytokines. The cytokines act as a signal to our body to send extra white blood cells and nutrients to aid in healing. Prostaglandins, which are a substance similar to hormones, trigger the pain and fever as well as create blood clots to help repair any damaged tissue. As the body heals, the inflammation will gradually lessen until no longer needed.

While acute inflammation is very useful in aiding the body to repair itself, chronic inflammation can cause more damage rather than repair it. Chronic inflammation is usually a low level throughout the entire body. It is often found by a small rise of immune system markers in blood or tissue samples.

Chronic inflammation can be caused by anything your body thinks is a threat, whether it really is or not. This inflammation will still trigger the white blood cells to respond, but because there is nothing that needs their attention to heal, they sometimes begin to attack healthy cells, tissues, and organs. While researchers are still trying to fully understand exactly how chronic inflammation works, it is known to increase the likelihood of developing many diseases.

Cases of acute inflammation are often easily treated with over the counter medications. Commonly used NSAID drugs and pain relievers like naproxen, ibuprofen, and aspirin are usually considered safe and effective against short term inflammation. These drugs work by blocking the enzyme cyclooxygenase, which produces the prostaglandins; this reduces the pain making it more bearable. If the over the counter medications do not ease the discomfort, there are prescription medications that may work as well, such as cortisone and steroids such as prednisone that are known to reduce inflammation. Unfortunately, there still are no medications specifically for treating chronic inflammation.

While there are many options to treat inflammation short term, all of the medications come with side effects and may not be safe to use long term.

NSAIDs, when used often over months or years time, can raise the risk of stroke or heart attack as well as stomach and bowel side effects such as ulcers and bleeding. Cortisone can cause weight gain, osteoporosis, diabetes, and muscle weakness. Prednisone is prescribed to treat a wide array of symptoms and diseases, but it can also suppress the immune system, causing an increased risk of infection. With long term use, it may also increase the risk of osteoporosis, thinning skin, fluid retention, and weight gain caused by increased hunger.

Medications may act quickly and help reduce the pain for a few hours, but they come with many risks and have to be taken daily, most often multiple times a day for continued relief. When inflammation becomes chronic and is affecting your daily life, it's time to begin looking for a safer long term solution to the inflammation. It may be just as easy as changing what and when you eat.

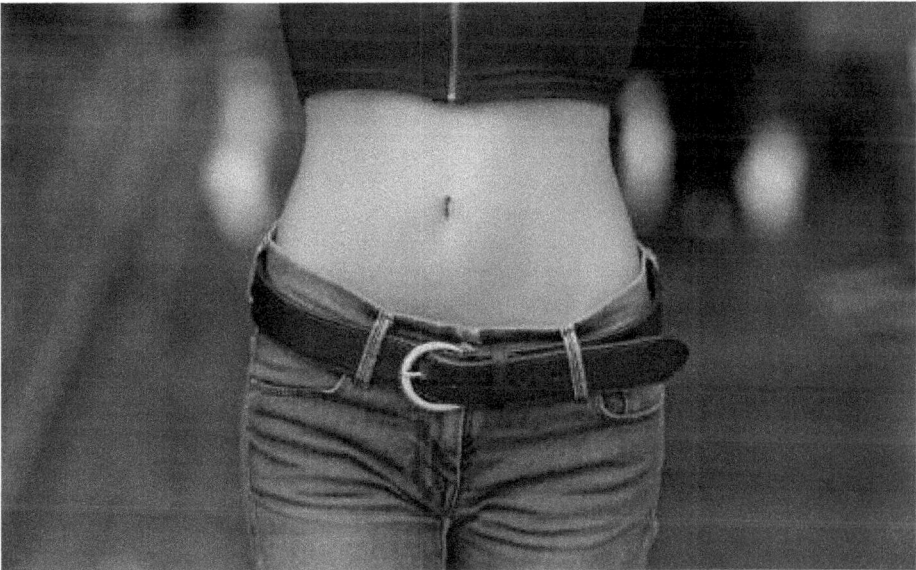

Chapter 2: Disease Prevention

Researchers are still trying to understand the specifics of inflammation and what the effects are on the body, but what is known is inflammatory foods are linked to a higher risk of long term and difficult to manage diseases like type 2 diabetes and heart disease.

Eating anti-inflammatory foods will calm your overactive immune system. By changing your way of eating you will not only reduce your symptoms of inflammation but you may even be able to reverse the progress of conditions you already have including inflammatory bowel and Crohn's disease, depression, anxiety, autoimmune diseases such as lupus, psoriasis, and types of arthritis, cardiovascular diseases, metabolic disorders such as diabetes, high cholesterol, asthma and even skin conditions such as eczema.

While large-scale studies are still needed, chronic inflammation has been linked to many major diseases that affect a large portion of society. Heart disease, arthritis, diabetes, Alzheimer's depression, and even cancers have been linked to inflammation. In experimental studies, it was found that there are many foods that have anti-inflammatory effects. These studies have also been able to pinpoint many of the foods and beverages that can cause inflammation to flare up.

By choosing the right foods to eat, you can lessen the inflammation in your body, slow down, or even cause current ailments to regress.

It is not surprising that the majority of foods found to cause inflammation are the foods that we have always been told are "unhealthy." We already know that eating too many unhealthy foods can cause us to gain weight, and additional weight can increase our risk of inflammation, but even when obesity was taken into account, there was still an undeniable link between foods and inflammation.

Chapter 3: A New Way of Life, A New You

You have the power to take control of your health. The Anti-Inflammatory Diet works to remove toxins and chemicals from the body that come from the average diet. While it will not work within an hour or two like pain medication will, it will reduce your chronic inflammation, increase your energy, and doesn't come with all of the side effects.

When living with chronic inflammation, are you really living? When fighting off chronic inflammation, you endure many symptoms that can change the way you live your life. You may find yourself going out less often due to pain or fatigue. You see, the world passing you by and may miss out on time that could have been spent with friends or grandchildren. As muscles and joints become stiff from swelling, you may move around less often, even in your own home. This often causes weight gain, which will only exacerbate the pain and inflammation. By consuming anti-inflammatory foods, you can reduce your pain and swelling within a matter of days. Once your inflammation is reduced, you will be up and moving around again in no time and be able to spend time playing with grandkids or going for a walk. You will feel the increase in your energy and know you were able to make those changes to your life by just eating healthy foods and knowing which foods to avoid.

It may seem difficult to give up so many of your favorite foods or to stick to a limited diet, but the benefits outweigh the losses. By letting go of the foods that cause inflammation, you will truly be able to take control of your life and your health. You will find that if you are strict and only eat anti-inflammatory foods, your taste buds will change, and so will your cravings. Soon you will not miss those sugary desserts, and you will find new favorites. Once you see and feel the difference as the inflammation subsides, you won't look back.

Inflammation can affect you in many different ways. You may not have even realized you were not feeling your best. It may just be your normal, and you didn't even know you could feel stronger or faster. You may have assumed it was natural due to aging or lack of sleep. You will find that once you begin the Anti-Inflammatory Diet, your fatigue will subside, and you will be able to sleep more soundly at night.

But for lasting health, you have to go into this not thinking of it as a diet, but truly as a new way of eating, a new way of life. While inflammation can be reduced by eating the correct foods, it can just as quickly come back if you fall back into your old eating habits. You have to be ready for this change. If you're sick of feeling sick and sore every day, you are the only one that can change that.

There currently are no long term medications to reduce chronic inflammation. You may be prescribed medications that treat some of the symptoms of inflammation, but many of those medications have side effects and can be hard on your liver and kidneys. These side effects may become so difficult to live with that you are now prescribed additional medications to treat the side effects of the first medication. It becomes a constant battle trying to get in front of it, and the cost of medications and doctor's visits only makes it more frustrating and causes additional stress in your life.

Make the decision to change your life for the better, eat healthy anti-inflammatory foods, even more importantly, STOP EATING INFLAMMATORY FOODS, and you will see less need for those doctor visits and medication.

Chapter 4: Foods Allowed/Avoid

Your diet can greatly impact your immune system. The micro biome (bacteria and microorganisms) in your digestive tract help to regulate your body's natural defense system. Everything you choose to eat will either cause inflammation or reduce it.

Choosing to consume a diet that consists of balanced fatty acids will help stifle low-grade chronic inflammation and enable you to feel your best. A basic anti-inflammatory diet focuses on removing sugary, processed foods and adding in high quantities of fresh produce, healthy fats, whole, unprocessed grains, spices, and herbs. It is also important to limit carbohydrates as they cause a great amount of inflammation, as well.

Colorful vegetables are known to be a good source of antioxidants. By adding a great array of colorful vegetables and eliminating the starchy ones, you will help support your immune system.

Legumes are another great source of antioxidants and protein. To cut down on additives, try choosing dried beans and just soak them overnight before rinsing and cooking.

Grains can be helpful in reducing inflammation by supplying fiber and antioxidants if you choose the correct ones. Many people are sensitive to gluten, even those who do not have celiac disease; this can cause digestive and systemic inflammation. Be sure to choose gluten-free unprocessed grains such as whole oats, quinoa, barley, and brown rice.

Extra Virgin Olive Oil is a great healthy fat and should be your go-to when cooking a meal or dressing a salad. Extra Virgin Olive Oil supplies monounsaturated fat, which can be good for your heart as well as antioxidants and a compound called oleocanthal that is known to lower inflammation.

While there are many foods that should be included in your diet to aid in reducing chronic inflammation, there are also some foods that you must avoid to help keep the inflammation down.

Processed foods and sugars are two of the biggest culprits when it comes to inflammation in the western diet. Processed foods are highly refined, causing them to lose much of their natural fiber and nutrients. They also are often high in omega 6, trans fats, and saturated fats, which all increase inflammation.

Sugar is one of the worst offenders when it comes to increased inflammation. Not only does it hide in many foods, studies have found that it is very addictive. Because of this, you should expect to go through a withdrawal phase when you remove it from your diet. This can often cause headaches, cravings, and sluggishness. Give yourself some time to allow your body to work through it. Sugar, even natural sugars such as honey and agave, cause the body to release cytokines, which causes an immune response leading to inflammation. You don't have to fully remove natural sugars from your diet, but you should work towards only eating them a few times a week and at no more than one meal per day.

Most fried foods, especially deep-fried foods, should be avoided as well. Usually, they are cooked in processed oils or lard and are coated in a refined flour that promotes inflammation.

You will want to pay attention to foods known as nightshades. Nightshades can be anti-inflammatory, but some people are sensitive to them, if you find you seem to have more inflammation after consuming a nightshade, you may want to begin to make substitutions in your recipes.

Below are many of the foods to increase in your diet as well as ones you should limit or avoid. This list is not all-inclusive, so remember to stick to the above points.

Foods to Enjoy		Foods to Avoid
Vegetables		**Vegetables**
Kale	String	Nightshades such as
Beans		Banana Peppers
Spinach	Water	Chili Peppers
Chestnut		Thai Peppers
Collards	Cauliflower	Tomatoes
Arugula	Fennel	Tomatillos
Broccoli	Lettuce	Pimentos
Carrots	Peppers	Sweet Peppers
Cabbage	Rhubarb	Habanero
Artichoke	Shallots	Eggplant
Asparagus		Jalapeno
Mushrooms		Potatoes (sweet potatoes are
Beets	Garlic	ok)
Brussel SproutsOnion		Artichoke
Zucchini Leeks		All canned and frozen
Squash Radishes		vegetables should be avoided.
Watercress Chard		
BeetsBok Choy		
Celery Cucumber		
Turnips		
		Fruits
		All canned and frozen fruits
Fruits		should be avoided.

Apple	Blueberries	
Watermelon		
Pomegranate		
Apricot	Cantaloupe	
Banana	Plum	
Strawberries	Pineapple	
Blackberries	Cherries	
Starfruit	Pear	
Dates	Papaya	
Figs	Orange	
Nectarine	Grapes	
Mango	Guava	
Lemon	Honeydew	
Kiwi	Clementine	

Vegetarian Protein

		Vegetarian Protein
Tempeh	Soy Nuts	Dairy
Edamame	Soy Milk	Frozen or processed meals
Tofu	Organic Eggs	Nonorganic eggs

Protein

		Protein
Tuna	Flounder	Red meat with hormones
Clams	Shrimp	Processed meats such as deli
Striped Bass	Rainbow Trout	meat, hot dogs, bacon, and
Snapper	Sardines	sausage.
Crab	Halibut	
Herring	Salmon	

Lobster Oysters Skinless Chicken Organic Eggs	
Grains Barley Black Rice Wild Rice Quinoa Brown Rice Oats Buckwheat Millet Bulgar Farro Corn	**Grains** White Rice Wheat Flour Corn
Starchy Vegetables Acorn Squash Yams Jicama Butternut Squash Gold Potatoes Parsnips Red Potatoes Artichoke Sweet Potatoes Pumpkin Purple Potatoes White Potatoes	**Starchy Vegetables** White Potatoes may cause inflammation for those sensitive to nightshades.
Fats and Oils Almonds Avocado Oil Almond Butter Cashews Almond Oil Cashew Butter	**Fats and Oils** Vegetable Oil Safflower Oil Soybean Oil Grape seed Oil

Olive Oil Hazelnuts WalnutsChia Seeds Walnut Oil Sesame Seed Oil Hemp seeds Flax Seeds Avocado Brazil Nuts Pumpkin Seeds Pecans Macadamia Nuts Olives Sunflower Seed Butter	Peanut Butter Mayonnaise Corn Oil
Herbs and Spices Turmeric Garlic Ginger Cinnamon Basil Thyme Black Pepper Sage Cilantro Parsley Cayenne Pepper Oregano Dill Mint Cloves Cumin	Cayenne Pepper and Chili Pepper may cause inflammation to those sensitive to nightshades.
Beverages Water Tea-Green, Black, White, Herbal, and Oolong	**Beverages** All other beverages should be avoided.
Nightshade Substitutions	

White Potato- Sweet Potato, Parsnips, or Turnips. Tomatoes- Beets, Pumpkin or Butternut Squash. Bell Peppers- Carrots, Celery, Cucumbers, or Radishes. Chili and Cayenne Pepper- Turmeric, Black Pepper, Cloves, Ginger or Garlic Powder. Eggplant- Portobello Mushrooms, Zucchini, or Okra.	

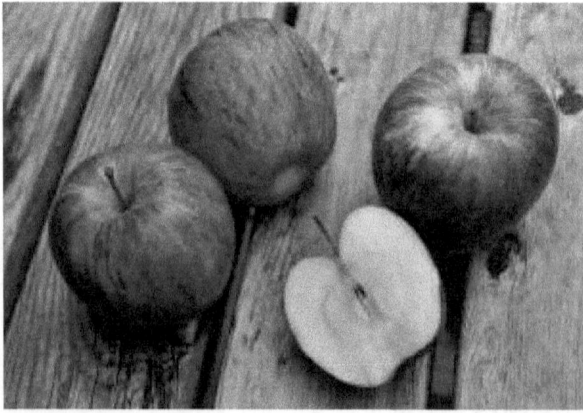

Chapter 5:3 Week Diet Plan

Now that you have a better understanding of what causes chronic inflammation in your body, it's time to start your new life. Included is enough recipes to get you through the next 21 days.

Breakfast Recipes

Coconut Flour Pancakes

Coconut flour - .25 Cup

Coconut milk - .25 Cup

Cold-pressed coconut oil – 2 Full tbsp

Organic eggs - 3

Honey – 2 Tbsp

Pure vanilla extract - .5 Tsp

A dash of baking soda

Salt - .0625 Tsp

Maple syrup to your preference

Grass-fed butter

Mix the honey, eggs, and coconut oil. Whisk until well mixed.

Next, add the coconut milk and vanilla extract into the egg mixture and combine.

Slowly pour in the salt, flour, and baking soda. Stir until well mixed but be careful; mixing too much will result in flat pancakes. It is recommended that you leave a couple of lumps in the mix.

Now, melt a little butter in your pan and add some batter using a ladle or measuring cup for easy pouring.

You won't see many bubbles in this batter as it is cooking, so you will need to carefully check the bottom of your pancake to make sure it is browned before flipping.

Finish cooking the other side of your pancake and serve with maple syrup.

If unhappy with the consistency of the pancakes, try adding another egg.

Makes 8 pancakes (depending on size) Serves 2.

Spinach and Kale Sweet Potato Cakes

Sweet potatoes – 2 Medium

Chopped spinach - .5 Cup

Kale - .5 Cup, chopped with stems removed

White onion - .25 Cup, finely chopped

Sea salt - .5 Tsp

Cumin – 1 Tsp

Avocado oil – 3 Tsp

Powdered garlic – 1 Tsp

Full fat coconut milk – 2 Tbsp

First, peel your potatoes and cut into cubes about ½ inch in size.

Add about 1 inch of water to a saucepan and using a steam basket, steam the potatoes until soft.

Once soft, move the sweet potatoes to a bowl. Add the milk and mash together until lumps are removed.

Next, add in the kale, onion, spinach, cumin, sea salt, and garlic. Stir until well combined.

Once combined, make 6-8 individual patties out of the mixture.

Warm avocado oil and then fry all patties until both sides have browned.

Makes 6 servings.

Turmeric Chocolate Chia Pudding

Coconut milk- 1 Can
Chia seeds-.33 Cups
Unsweetened cacao powder-.25 Cups
Cinnamon-.5 Tsp
Ground turmeric-1 Tsp
Raw honey -.5 Tbsp
Vanilla extract-.5 Tsp

Toppings: you may choose nuts, fruit, shredded coconut, etc.

Add vanilla, honey, turmeric, cinnamon, cacao powder, chia seeds and milk to a blender and blend together until a smooth consistency has been reached.

Store the mixture in the fridge, covered, for at least 4 hours until it thickens.

Pour into bowl and add desired toppings.

Serve chilled.

Makes 2 servings.

Mango Turmeric Overnight Oats

Rolled oats-.5 Cup

Milk kefir or Greek yogurt-.5 Cup

Almond milk-.5 Cup

Maple syrup-2 Tsp

Ground turmeric-.25 Tsp

Cardamom-.25 Tsp

Chia seeds-1 Tbsp

Ground cinnamon-.25 Tsp

Ginger-.25 Tsp

Finely chopped mango (fresh or frozen)-Half

Using 2 mason jars, add ¼ cup of rolled oats, ¼ cup of milk kefir or Greek yogurt, and ¼ cup of almond milk to each jar.

Divide the chia seeds and spices between the jars. Stir until well combined.

Top the jars with the finely chopped mango.

Refrigerate jars overnight.

Enjoy cold straight from the jar or pour into a bowl and heat in the microwave.

Makes 2 servings.

Maple Rice Porridge Bake

Brown rice-.5 Cup
Vanilla extract-.5 Tsp
Pure maple syrup-2 Tbsp
A pinch of cinnamon
A small dash of salt (optional)
Sliced fruit such as pears, plums, berries or cherries

Turn the oven on to bake at 400 degrees Fahrenheit and allow it to preheat.

Pour the rice and one cup of the water into a saucepan and warm to boiling on a medium/high heat.

Onceitis boiling, drop in the cinnamon and vanilla extract then stir until well combined.

Place a cover on the pot and turn down the heat to a medium/low.

For 10-15 minutes, let the rice simmer until it is tender.

Stir the rice and divide into two oven-safe serving containers. Add maple syrup and desired sliced fruit to the top each bowl, and sprinkle with salt is desired.

Bake the rice bowls for about 10-15 minutes until the syrup begins to bubble, and the fruit topping just starts to caramelize.

Serve immediately.

Makes 2 servings.

Pecan Banana Overnight Oats

Old fashioned rolled oats-1 Cup
Ripe bananas-2 Mashed

Almond milk-1.5 Cups

Plain Greek yogurt-.25 Cup

Chia seeds- Tbsp

Honey-2 Tbsp

Unsweetened coconut flakes-2 Tbsp toasted

Vanilla extract-2 Tsp

Flaked sea salt-.25 Tsp

Banana slices, fig halves, roasted pecans, pomegranate seeds, and honey for serving

Mix the ingredients together (except or the fruit and nuts for serving).

Mix together, so the items are blended thoroughly.

Split the mix evenly between 2 bowls or glass jars.

Place a cover over the bowls and allow to cool in the fridge overnight or for a minimum of 6 hours.

Stir the mixture and then heat up the mixture if desired.

Top with the banana slices, figs, roasted pecans, and pomegranate seeds. Drizzle with honey and enjoy.
Makes 2 servings.

Breakfast Bowl

Whole grains like amaranth or buckwheat-1 Cup

Nut milk or coconut water-2.5 Cups

Cinnamon-1 Stick

Whole cloves-2

Star anise (optional)-1 Pod

Fresh fruits such as cranberries, blackberries, apples, pears, or any others you prefer

Maple syrup (optional)

Pour the grains, coconut water or nut milk and spices into a small pot and warm over a mid-level to high heated burner until boiling.

Once the grains are boiling, cover the saucepan and turn down the burner to a mid-level to low. Let the grains simmer until they are tender, usually about 20-25 minutes.

Discard the whole spices and take the pan off of the stovetop.

Top with a little maple syrup and your fruit of choice.

Makes 2 servings.

Turkey Apple Hash

For the meat:

Ground turkey-1 Pound

Cinnamon-.5 Tsp

Dried thyme-.5 Tsp

Coconut oil-1 Tbsp

Sea salt to taste

For the hash:

Carrots-.5 Cups shredded

Coconut oil-.5 Tbsp

Zucchini-1 Large

Onion-1

Apple-1 Large, peeled, cored and chopped into small cubes

Butternut squash-2 Cups frozen, cut into cubes

Spinach- 2 Cups

Powdered Ginger-.75 Tsp

Cinnamon-1 Tsp

Powdered garlic-.5 Tsp

Turmeric-.5 Tsp

Dried thyme-.5 Tsp

Sea salt if desired

Warm the coconut oil over a mid-level to high heated burner.

Cook the turkey and cook until it browns.

Add .5 tsp of cinnamon, thyme, and salt to the ground turkey to season. Mix in, then move to a plate.

Using the same skillet, add the remaining coconut oil and use it to saute the onion until it softens.

To the skillet, add the apple, carrots, zucchini, and frozen squash and cook for about 4.5 minutes. Once the vegetables become soft, stirin the spinach
until it wilts.

Next, add the cooked turkey and the remainder of the seasonings to the skillet, mix until well combined. Sprinkle in some salt if needed and turn the cook top off.

Enjoy the hash fresh and hot or store it in the fridge to save for later.

When stored in a well-sealed container, the hash will stay fresh for about 5-6 days in the refrigerator.

Makes 5 servings.

Chia Energy Bar

Pitted dates–1.5 Cups packed

Raw walnut pieces – 1.25 Cups

Raw cacao powder-.33 Cup

Whole chia seeds-.5 Cup

Unsweetened coconut-.5 Cups, shredded

Whole oats-.5 Cup

Pure vanilla extract-1 Tsp

Dark chocolate-.5 Cup chopped

Sea salt-.25 Tsp

Puree the dates in a processing appliance until they become thick and smooth.

Add raw walnut pieces to the blender and mix well.

Pour in the rest of the ingredients, mix together.

Once it reaches a dough-like consistency, use a piece of parchment paper to line a square baking pan leaving a few extra inches above the pan to make it easy to remove and press the dough into the pan firmly so that it fills to all corners.

Place the baking pan into the freezer overnight or at the least, 4 hours.

Take the pan from the freezer and lift the mixture out of the pan.

Use a knife to cut into 14 bars.

Can be stored in an airtight container in the fridge.

Makes 14 servings.

Banana Chia Pudding

Banana-1 Large
Chia seeds-.5 Cup
Raw honey-2 Tbsp
Unsweetened almond milk-2 Cups
Vanilla extract- .5 Tsp
Cacao powder-1 Tbsp

Mix ins:

Banana-1 Large

Dark chocolate chips-2 Tbsp

Cacao nibs-2 Tbsp

In a medium bowl, mash together a banana and the chia seeds using a fork until combined well.

Add almond milk and vanilla extract, use your whisk and combine until there are no more lumps.

Pour half of your mixture into a covered, airtight container.

Add the honey (or maple syrup) and cacao powder to the remaining half and whisk again until combined.

In a second container, pour the cacao mixture and cover. Place the two containers into the fridge overnight or for at least 4 hours.

To serve, layer the two puddings and mix-ins into 3 separate containers in even layers.

Can be refrigerated in a well-sealed bowl for up to 5 days.

Makes 3 servings.

Porridge

Walnut or pecan halves- .25 Cup roughly chopped

Unsweetened toasted coconut- .25 Cup

Hemp seeds-2 Tablespoons

Unsweetened almond milk- .75 Cups

Whole chia seeds-2 Tablespoons

Coconut milk- .25 Cup

Coconut oil-3 Tsp

Cinnamon - .5 Tsp

Almond butter- .25 Cup

Powdered turmeric- .5 Tsp

Black pepper- .0625 Tsp

Roast the chopped walnuts (or pecans), coconut, and hemp seeds in a heated pan for about 1-2 minutes until fragrant. Toss the coconut and nuts a few times to keep them from burning in the pan.

Pour the nuts onto a plate and put to the side until no longer hot.

Warm the almond and coconut milk in a small saucepan on a mid-level to high heated burner.

Once the milk become warm, but not yet boiling, take them off of the burner.

Stir the cinnamon and turmeric powder together and add to the milk along with the coconut oil, almond butter, chia seeds, and black pepper. Mix together until well combined and set aside for about 5-8 minutes to cool slightly.

Include about half of the seed and nut mix and stir in.

Split the porridge between two bowls and sprinkle the remaining roasted mix over the top.

Immediately serve or store in the refrigerator in a well-sealed bowl for no longer than 3 days. If storing, keep the remaining roasted mix separate and store at room temperate. Add just before serving to keep the crunch.

Makes 2 servings.

<u>Sweet Potato Muffins</u>

Cooked sweet potato-1 Small

Organic egg-1

Brown rice flour-1 Cup

Coconut milk- .75 Cup

Coconut flour- .25 Cup

Pure maple syrup- .5 Cup

Baking powder-3 Tsp

Olive oil-6 Tsp

Salt-1/2 Tsp

Powdered cinnamon-3 Tsp

Powdered ginger-1 Tsp

Powdered turmeric-1 Tsp

Ground cloves- .125 Tsp

Ground nutmeg- .125 Tsp

Turn oven on to bake at 400 degrees Fahrenheit.

Once cooked, allow the sweet potato to cool and cut it in two. Scoop the insides of the sweet potato into a bowl using a spoon.

Add egg, olive oil, maple syrup, and coconut milk and mix together with the sweet potato until smooth.

In a separate bowl, combine all remaining items and then pour them into the sweet potato. Stir until well combined.

Grease your muffin pan and evenly pour the batter until each muffin cup filled about 2/3 of the way.

low-grade

Makes 12 servings.

Turmeric Oven Baked Eggs

Organic eggs – 8 to 10 Large

Unsweetened almond milk- .5 Cup

Black pepper- .25 Tsp

Powdered turmeric- .75 Tsp

A pinch of cumin

Sea salt - .25 Tsp

At least 2-inch deep sheet pan (about 18" x 26" or a 9" x 13" baking pan)

Optional toppings- avocado, salsa, cilantro, etc.

Turn the oven on and allow it to heat to 350 degrees Fahrenheit

Use a whisk to combine the eggs, milk, and spices in a medium-sized bowl.

Oil the sheet pan (or baking pan).

Gently pour the eggs onto the sheet pan.

Put the eggs in the oven for 10 to 12 minutes to bake. Once eggs have started to set, take them out of the oven and gently stir the eggs, being careful not to spill any, then place the pan back into the oven.

Keep baking the eggs for another 8 to 10 minutes or until eggs are set.

Remove eggs from oven and stir again.

Serve the eggs as is or top with peppers, cilantro, avocado, etc.

Baked eggs can also be stored for up to 4 days in a refrigerated airtight container.

If you want to use the eggs for an easy sandwich, you can also allow them to bake for about 15 to 17 minutes without stirring and then slice into squares.

Makes 5-6 servings.

Berry and Turmeric Muffins

Whole wheat flour – 1.33 Cups
Coconut oil- .5 Cup plus additional to grease the tins
All-purpose flour–8 Ounces
Sugar in the Raw- .5 Cup
Unsweetened almond milk–8 Ounces
Maple syrup- .33 Cup plus 1 Tbsp

Baking soda-1 Tsp

Baking powder - 1 Tsp

Turmeric-.5 Tbsp

Salt- .5 Tsp

Cardamom- .5 Tsp

Pure vanilla extract- .5 Tsp

Organic eggs-2 at room temperature, beaten

Apple cider vinegar-2 Tsp

Chopped walnuts-1 Cup

Fresh or frozen raspberries-1 Cup

Chia seeds-1 tbsp

Fresh or frozen blueberries-1 Cup

Rolled oats-3 Tbsp

Turn the oven on to bake at 400 degrees Fahrenheit.

Use coconut oil to cover 2 muffin tins.

Whisk together the all-purpose flour, whole wheat flour, salt, baking powder, baking soda, turmeric, and cardamom until mixed completely.

Using another bowl, combine sugar and coconut oil for about 1 to 2 minutes so that the sugar dissolves a bit. Then add the maple syrup, almond milk, eggs, vanilla extract, and stir in the apple cider vinegar until well combined.

Fold together the dry ingredients and the egg mixture until they are well combined but leaving some small lumps.

Gently add in the berries, walnuts, and chia seeds.

Fill the muffin tins with the batter until about 2 to 3 full and add some rolled oats and remaining sugar in the raw to the tops.

Let the muffin batter rest for about 5 minutes.

Put the muffins into the oven and cook for 13 to 15 minutes. Test muffins to see if they are done by sticking a wooden toothpick directly into the middle of one of the muffins if it is clean when taken out the muffins are done.

Removing muffins and place them on a cooling rack after allowing them to stay in the pan to cool for 10 minutes.

Makes 18 servings.

Pumpkin Pancakes

Pumpkin puree- .25 Cup

Very ripe banana-1

Coconut flour- .5 Cup

Coconut oil-3 Tablespoons melted

Ground cinnamon- .5 Tsp

Organic eggs–4

Black pepper - .125 Tsp

Pure vanilla extract-1 Tsp

Ground turmeric-.75 Tsp

Your choice of cooking oil

Add everything but the cooking oil to a blender, mix well, stopping to scrape the side to ensure it is well combined.

Give the batter a few minutes to rest to allow the liquid to be absorbed by the coconut flour.

Turn on the cook top to a medium heat and allow a skillet to heat, then add your cooking oil.

Once your skillet is hot, carefully pour the batter to make pancakes about 3" in diameter.

Cook for a minute or two to allow to lightly brown, then flip and repeat on the other side.

Serve warm and top with maple syrup, honey, or fresh fruit.

Makes 10-12 small pancakes.

Zuppe and Stews

Vegetable Soup

Water – 3 or 4 Cups

Cauliflower florets- 3 Cups chopped

Great Northern Beans-15Ounces, canned drain then rinsed

Shirataki noodles-1 7 ounce package, drained

Kale-1 Bunch, chopped

Vegetable broth-1 32 ounce carton

Diced onion-1

Carrot-1 Medium, cut fine

Olive oil-1 Tbsp

Celery-2 Stalks, cut fine

Ground turmeric-1 Tbsp

Ground ginger- .5 Tsp

Minced Garlic-2 Tsp

Ground cayenne pepper- .25 Tsp

Salt – 1 Tsp

A pinch of black pepper

Heat the oil over a mid-level to low heated burner.

To the pot, add onion and allow to cook while stirring until brown.

Next, celery and carrots should be added to the pot to soften, mixing often.

Stir in the turmeric, ginger, garlic, and cayenne to evenly coverall of the veggies. Cook for about 1 minute until you can smell the flavors combining.

Add the water, broth, salt, and pepper then stir until well mixed.

Allow the pot to boiling, then turn the burner down to a low setting so that it just simmers.

Add the chopped cauliflower and cover the pot. Allow to simmer for about 10 to 15 minutes until the cauliflower softens.

Once cauliflower has softened some, the beans, kale, and noodles can be added to the pot.

Cook until the kale has wilted slightly and serve hot.

Makes 4 servings.

Cream of Broccoli Soup

Ghee or grass-fed butter-3 Tsp

White onion- .5 Diced

Garliccloves-2, minced

Chicken or bone broth-3 Cups

Coconut milk–8 Ounces

Broccoli florets-1 Pound

Leek-1 (whites only)

Pepper and saltas needed

Heat the ghee over a mid-level to high heated burner.

Cook the onion in the ghee for about 1 to 2 minutes and soft and translucent.

Next, cook the garlic with onion, stirring often for 1 minute.

Carefully, pour the leeks, broth, and broccoli to the pot and add pepper and saltas needed.

Allow the pot to boil for a minute or so before lowering the heat to simmer the broccoli for about 20 minutes; the broccoli should be tender.

Coconut milk can then be added to the pot. Allow the milk to fully warm and then move all the ingredients from the pot to a food processing appliance. Puree until the soup no longer has lumps, and it well combined.

Transfer to bowls and serve immediately.

Serve hot.

Makes 4-6 servings.

Shrimp Bisque

Red bell pepper-1 Large
Light coconut milk-15 Ounces
Chicken broth-2 Cups
Minced Garlic-1 Tsp
BBQ sauce- .25 Cup
Shallots- .75 Cup, chopped
Olive oil-3 Tsp

Water-3 Tsp

Tapioca or potato starch-2 Tbsp

Ground mustard - .25 Tsp

Cayenne- .5 Tsp

Flaked red pepper-1 Tsp

A pinch of ground ginger

Fresh cilantro for garnish

Turn oven on to bake at 475 degrees Fahrenheit.

Roast the red pepper for 10 minutes on a sheet pan. Rotate the pepper and continue cooking for about 5 to 10 minutes longer.

Broil pepper on low for the last 2 to 3 minutes.

Remove the sheet pan from the oven to cool.

Once cooled, the pepper skin can be taken off the pepper, then slice the stem off of the top and remove the seeds.

In a medium-sized pot, sauté the minced garlic and shallots in the oil over amid-level heated burner.

Once the flavors have been released, pour the water and peeled shrimp into the pot.

Allow the shrimp to cook at a medium heat until all are pink, about 6 to 8 minutes for medium-sized shrimp.

Add in black pepper and salt and stir to combine.

Take the shrimp out of the pot and set aside once cooked.

Pour the coconut milk, broth, starch, and seasonings to the pot and stir well to combine.

Mix the ingredients while simmering for about 5 minutes.

Blend the roasted pepper, liquid, and BBQ sauce in a blender until creamy.

Transfer the bisque back to the pot until it reaches a low boil. Turn down the burner to an until simmering and allow to cook for 10 to 20 minutes before returning the shrimp to the bisque.

Return the shrimp back to the bisque.

Serve immediately and garnish with fresh cilantro.

Makes 4 servings.

Mexican Chicken Soup

Fire-roasted plum tomatoes-1 14 ounce can

Boneless, skinless, chicken breast-1 Pound

Red bell pepper-1 Chopped

Half and half-1 Cup

Chicken stock – 1.5 Cups

Cream cheese- .5 Cup room temperature

Cheddar cheese-1 cup shredded

Olive oil-2 Tsp

Garlic-1 Tbsp minced

Onion - 1 Medium, diced

Paprika - 1 Tsp

Powdered cumin – 1.5 Tsp

Chipotle chili powder – .5 Tbsp

Dried oregano-1 Tsp

Salt to taste

Fresh cilantro for garnish

Warm the oil over a mid-level heated burner.

Once the oil is heated, fry together the onion and the garlic, stirring often to keep them from burning. Remove from the heat once softened.

In a preheated slow cooker, add the chicken breast, fire-roasted tomatoes, onion, garlic, all spices, and chicken stock. Add salt to taste.

Heat in your slow cooker on a high setting for 3 hours.

Mix in chopped bell pepper, cream cheese, half and half, and shredded cheese. Heat, covered for an additional 20 minutes to a half an hour for the cheeses to become melted.

Once done, using 2 forks, shred the chicken and stir the soup again until combined.

Top soup with fresh cilantro, or avocado and sour cream when serving.

Makes 5 servings.

Miso Soup

Water-4 Cups
Fish stock-1 Cup
Shiitake mushrooms-6 Dried
Potatoes-2 Large, cubed
Kombu-1 Piece
Yellow onion-1 Finely chopped
Firm tofu-1 Block, cubed
Carrot-1 Thinly sliced
Brown miso paste-2 Tbsp
Dried wakame-2 Tbsp
White miso paste-1 Tbsp
Chopped green onion for garnish

Allow the dried shiitake mushrooms to soak for about 10 minutes in warm water. Drain the mushrooms and set the liquid aside for later. Slice the mushrooms.

Pour the water and potatoes into a large pot. Bring the water to boiling over a mid-level to high heated burner.

Reduce the heated burner to a low setting and continue cooking. Once the potatoes are just becoming easy to be pierced with a fork, add the yellow onion, fish stock, kombu, tofu, sliced shiitake mushrooms, carrot, and wakame and cook in the pot until all veggies are done.

Add both miso pastes to the soup and mash them until they completely dissolve.

Serve soup garnished with the green onions.

Makes 2 servings.

Red Lentil and Squash Stew

Broth-4 Cups
Red lentils-1 Cup
Choice of greens-1 Cup
Butternut squash- 3 Cups cooked
Extra virgin olive oil-1 Tsp
Garlic cloves-3 , minced
Powdered curry-1 Tbsp
Sweet onion - 1 Chopped
Fresh grated ginger to taste
Black pepper and salt as needed

Saute the olive oil, chopped onion, and garlic in a large pot for around 5 minutes on a low to mid-level heated burner.

Mix in the powdered curry and allow to saute together and combine for 2 to 3 minutes.

Carefully pouring the broth, then the red lentil sallow stew to come to begin boiling.

Once the stew has begun to boil, turn the heat on the burner down and continue to cook for another 10 minutes or so.

Stir the cooked squash and greens into the stew and simmer for around 5 to 8 minutes on a mid-level heated burner, then season as needed with ginger, pepper, and salt.

Makes 4 servings.

Turkey Chili

Lean ground turkey-1 Pound
Red bell pepper-1 Chopped
Tomato sauce - 30Ounces, canned
Black beans–30 Ounces canned, drained then rinsed

Yellow bell pepper-1 Chopped

Petite diced tomatoes–30 Ounces, canned

Frozen corn-1 Cup

Red kidney beans–30 Ounces, canned drained and rinsed

Deli sliced jalapeno peppers-1 16 ounce jar

Onion-1 Medium, diced

Olive oil-3 Tsp

Cumin–3 Tsp

Chili powder-2 Tbsp

Pepper and salt

Optional Toppings: avocado, shredded cheese, sour cream, green onion

Warm the olive oil over a mid-level heated burner.

Cook the turkey in the skillet until brown, then transfer it to the crock of your slow cooker.

Place the tomato sauce, beans, onions, jalapenos, peppers, diced tomatoes, cumin, chili powder, and corn into the slow cooker, add pepper and salt.

Stir together the ingredients and place the cover over your cooker. Allow to heat for 6 hours on a low setting or for 4 hours on the high setting.

Makes 8 servings.

Beef and Sweet Potato Stew

Beef chuck roast-3 Pounds

Beef broth – 1.5 Cup

Diced tomatoes - 1 14 ounce can

Tomato paste- .25 Cup

Almond flour- .33 Cup

Onion-1 Large, chopped

Garlic-6 cloves, crushed

Sweet potato-3 cups, peeled and diced into 2" cubes

Baby potatoes- .66 Pounds, halved

Carrots- 2 Large, sliced

Red bell pepper-1 Deseeded and chopped

Beef bouillon cubes-2 Crushed

Olive oil-.25 Cup

Salt-1 Tsp

Black pepper- .5 Tsp

Bay leaves–2

Paprika - 1 Tsp

Parsley-4 Tbsp, fresh chopped for garnish

Sprinkle pepper and salt over all sides of the beef.

On a medium/high heat, in a frying pan, heat 1 tablespoon of oil.

Sear the beef for 2 to 3 minutes per side until browned. Cook in batches to not overcrowd the pan and add additional oil as needed.

Once the meat has been seared, move it to the crock of your slow cooker.

Using the oil leftover in the frying pan, cook the onion until just softened. Drop the garlic in with the onion and continue sautéing for around60 seconds.

Move the garlic and onion to the crock along with the beef.

Mix in the flour and cover the meat, garlic, and onion by stirring . Add all of the remaining ingredients, but the bay leaves and parsley on top. Stir the ingredients until well combined, then add in the bay leaves.

Place the cover onto the crock and heat for 4 to 6 hours on a high setting or for 8 to 10 hours on a low setting.

Add salt or pepper if needed and garnish using the parsley as serving.

Makes 8 servings.

Tomato, Kale and Quinoa Soup

Vegetable broth-4 Cups

Quinoa-1 Cup uncooked and rinsed

Water-2 Cups

Great Northern beans-1 15 ounce can rinsed then drained

Petite diced tomatoes-2 14.5 ounce cans

Garlic-3 cloves, minced

Dried basil - .5

Onion-1 Diced

Dried rosemary - .25 Tsp

Dried oregano- .5 Tsp

Bay leaves–2

Kale - 1 Bunch chopped, stems removed

Dried thyme - .25 Tsp

Ground black pepper and salt

In a slow cooker, add the quinoa, tomatoes, beans, garlic, onion, rosemary, basil, oregano, bay leaves, and thyme.

Pouring the broth and water and stir until combined well. Sprinkle in salt and pepper if needed.

Place the cover onto the crock of your slow cooker, allow to heat for 7 to 8 hours on a low setting or 3 to 4 hours on a high setting.

Add the kale and stir until wilted, then serve.

Makes 8 Servings.

Kale and Turkey Meatball Soup

Great Northern beans-1 15 ounce can drained then rinsed
Vegetable broth-8 Cups
Almond milk- .25 Cup
Parmesan- .5 Cup, grated
Bread-2 Slices
Carrots-2 Peeled and sliced

Yellow onion- .5 Chopped

Lean ground turkey-1 Pound

Kale-4 Cups

Organic egg-1 Beaten

Garliccloves-2, diced

Shallot-1 Medium, chopped fine

Grated nutmeg- .5 Tsp

Flaked red pepper- .25 Tsp

Oregano-1 Tsp

Olive oil-1 Tbsp

Italian parsley-2 Tbsp, chopped

Tear bread into chunks and allow to soak in a medium-sized bowl of milk.

Then add the garlic, ground turkey, nutmeg, shallot, pepper, red pepper flakes, oregano, cheese, parsley, egg, and salt, then using your hands, gently mix to combine all ingredients.

Form meat mixture into ½" balls.

Heat the oil in a large frying pan over a medium-high heat and lightly sear all of the meatballs for about 1 to 2 minutes on each side.

Remove the meatballs from the pan and set aside.

Add the broth, carrots, beans, kale, and onions to the slow cooker.

Put the meatballs into the slow cooker on top of the kale, cover, and cook on low for 4 hours until the meatballs float to the top.

Serve the soup garnished with grated parmesan and parsley.

Makes 8 servings.

Broccoli Soup

Broccoli – 8 Cup, florets
Stock – 6 Cups
Leeks – 4 Cups, chopped
Butter – 2 Tbsp
Ginger – 2 Tbsp
Ground turmeric – 1 Tsp
Salt – 1 Tsp
Sesame oil – 1 Tbsp
A pinch of ground black pepper

Melt the butter in a large frying pan over medium heat.

Add the leeks and cook while stirring occasionally for about 8 minutes, until the leeks are cooked.

Transfer the leeks to your slow cooker and add the stock, ginger, broccoli, turmeric, sesame oil, and salt.

Cover the slow cooker and cook on low for 3 to 4 hours until the broccoli is tender.

Using a blender, blend soup until it is smooth and creamy.

Makes 6-8 servings.

Chicken Zoodle Soup

Chicken – 4 Cups, cooked and chopped
Low sodium chicken broth – 6 Cups
Onions – 2 medium, diced
Garlic – 6 cloves, minced
Carrots – 3 Large, peeled and diced
Zucchini or prepackaged zoodles – 2 Medium
Celery – 3 Large stalks and leaves, diced

Avocado oil – 2 Tbsp

Ground turmeric – 1 Tbsp

Bay leaves - 3

Dried rosemary – 1 Tsp

Dried sage – 1 Tsp

Dried thyme – 1 Tsp

Sea salt – 1 Tsp plus more to taste

In a large pot, heat the avocado oil over a medium-high heat.

Add in the turmeric and allow to cook in the oil for about 90 seconds while stirring to help bring out the flavor.

Add in the onions and garlic and cook until just translucent, stirring occasionally.

Next, add in the celery and carrots and cook until the vegetables just begin to soften.

Carefully add the broth, chicken, sage, bay leaves, rosemary, thyme, and sea salt.

Bring soup to a boil, then reduce heat and allow to simmer, uncovered for 25 to 30 minutes.

Once vegetables are tender and chicken is falling apart, check for seasoning and add additional salt if needed.

Using a spiralizer with noodle attachment, spiralize to zucchinis. Use a knife to cut the zucchini noodles into 2" to 3" pieces. (If you do not have a spiralizer you can purchase prepackaged zoodles)

Take the pot of soup from the cook top and take the bay leaves out.

Add the zoodles in and stir well. The heat left in the soup will be enough to cook the zoodles until softened. Enjoy!

Makes 6-8 servings.

Cauliflower Turmeric Soup

Cauliflower-1 Medium head, chopped
Unsweetened almond milk/cashew milk blend – 2.5 Cups
Vegetable broth-2 Cups
Red lentils- .5 Cup
Shallot-1 Medium, quartered
Garlic-3 or 4Cloves

Turmeric-1 Tsp

Olive oil-6 Tsp

Sea salt- .5 Tsp

Powdered cumin-1 Tsp

Garnish with cracked pepper, lime, fresh herbs, etc.

Turn the oven on to bake at 425 degrees Fahrenheit.

Drizzle olive oil over the cauliflower, shallots, and garlic in a large mixing bowl.

Move the vegetables to roast for 15 minutes on a large baking sheet. Flip veggies over then roast for an additional 15 minutes.

Once vegetables are roasted, transfer them to a large saucepan.

Carefully pour in2 cups of milk, the broth, and lentils. Mix well until combined.

Allow the soup to boil then add a cover. Simmer for 20 minute sat a reduced heat.

Pour the soup into a blending appliance and mix. Once well combined and there are no longer any lumps, stir in the remaining milk and top with the desired garnish.

Makes 4 servings.

Creamy Lemon Chicken Soup

Bone broth-6 Cups
Chicken-4 Cups cooked and shredded
Olive oil- .5 Cup
Onion-1 Cup, diced
Kale-1 Bunch
Lemon juice-2 Tbsp, fresh
Lemons-3
Salt

Wash the kale, stack the leaves in 2 piles and slice into ½" strips, then set aside.

In a blender, add 2 cups of broth, olive oil, and diced onion. Blend for 1-2 minutes until smooth.

Pour the blender contents into your crockpot and add the remaining 4 cups of broth. Add the shredded chicken, chopped kale, and zest of all 3 lemons along with the fresh lemon juice. Add salt to taste.

Let the soup cook on low for 6 hours.

Makes 6 servings.

Colorful Vegetable Soup

Water-4 Cups

Butternut squash-2 Cups diced

Red bell pepper-2 cups diced

Celery stalk-2 Cups diced

Carrots-1 Cup diced

Zucchini-1 Cup diced

Red onion-1 Cup diced

Spring onions-1 Cup chopped plus additional for garnish

Celery leaves-1 Cup

Garlic- 3 Large Cloves

Lemon juice-2 Tbsp

Salt to taste

Combine the water, red bell pepper, butternut squash, zucchini, red onion, spring onion, celery leaves, stalks, and garlic cloves into a large pot.

Bring the water to a boil then lower to medium heat. Let the ingredients simmer for about 40 minutes until the vegetables are tender.

Once done, add in the lemon juice and mix well. Add salt to taste.

Makes 4 servings.

Salads and Sides

Beet Salad

Sweet Kale Salad Mix (comes with a nut and seed packet)-24-ounce bag
Beets-16 ounces, cooked, peeled and chopped
Blueberries – 1.5 Cups, fresh

Turmeric Dressing:
Extra virgin olive oil- .33 Cup
Lemon juice-1 Tbsp
Apple cider vinegar-2 Tbsp
Turmeric-1 Tsp
Grated ginger-1 Tsp, fresh
Garlic-1 Clove, grated
Sea salt- .5 Tsp
Ground black pepper- .25 Tsp

Mix together all of the dressing ingredients. You can shake them or blend them if you would like a smoother dressing.

Divide the kale salad mix between bowls and top with the blueberries, beets, and the nut and seed mixture.

Drizzle with the turmeric dressing.

Makes 4-6 servings.

Tuna Salad

Cannellini beans – 1 15 ounce can rinsed and drained
Oil packed tuna – 1 Can (Use 2 cans if you would like the salad
to be tuna heavy)
Onion - .5 Cup, diced
Parsley - .25 Cup, finely minced
Fresh herb such as basil – 1 or 2 Tbsp
Extra virgin olive oil to taste
Salt to taste
Freshly ground black pepper to taste
Red wine vinegar to taste

Rinse and drain the can of beans. Add them to a medium mixing
bowl.

Add the tuna to the beans. (Do not drain)

Add the onion to the tuna and beans and mix.

Add the minced parsley and basil and mix well.

Season with the salt and pepper and drizzle with the olive oil and red wine vinegar. Enjoy!

Makes 2 servings.

Quinoa Salad

Roasted Almonds:

Raw almonds- .33 Cup

Maple syrup-1 Tsp

Low sodium tamari-1 Tsp

Coconut oil-1 Tsp

Sea salt- .25tsp or to taste

Salad:

Quinoa-2 Cups cooked

Chickpeas-2 Cups cooked, rinsed and drained

Cucumber-2 Cups, diced

Edamame-1 Cup, shelled

Purple cabbage-1 Cup, shredded

Mixed bell peppers-1 Cup

Celery – 1.5 Cups, finely diced

Red onion- .25 Cup, diced

Parsley- .25 Cup, fresh chopped

Pumpkin seeds-2 Tbsp

Sunflower seeds- Tbsp

Sesame seeds-2 Tsp

Dressing:

Lime juice-2 Tbsp fresh

Tahini-2 Tbsp

Apple cider vinegar-3 Tbsp

Maple syrup- .5 Tsp

Salt and ground black pepper to taste

Preheat the oven to 375 degrees Fahrenheit.

Toss the almonds in maple syrup and tamari in a large bowl. Sprinkle with sea salt and drizzle the coconut oil over the almonds, then toss again.

Cover a baking sheet in foil and lay the almonds out evenly in a single layer.

Roast the almonds for about 15 to 20 minutes, stirring and flipping occasionally.

While the almonds are roasting, combine all the dressing ingredients into a jar, close tightly, and shake until well combined.

Once almonds are done roasting, transfer them to a plate or a bowl to allow to cool.

Using a large bowl, stir together all of the remaining salad ingredients. Pour some dressing over the top, add the cooled almonds and toss well.

Makes 11 small servings.

<u>Chickpea Salad</u>

Citrus Vinaigrette:
Fresh squeezed orange juice-2 Tbsp
Orange zest- .5 Tsp
Fresh squeezed lemon juice-1 Tbsp
Lemon zest- .5 Tsp
Fresh oregano-1 Tbsp, finely chopped
Olive oil-2 Tbsp
Mint leaves-2.5 Tbsp fresh, julienned
Salt to taste
Ground black pepper to taste

Salad:

Chickpeas-2 Cups, cooked and drained

Red bell pepper-1 Small, diced

Red onion- .5 Cup, diced

Cucumber-1 Medium, diced

Tomatoes-2 Medium, diced

Green olives (water-packed)- .25 Cup, drained

Pomegranates- .5 Cup

Add orange juice and zest, lemon juice and zest, olive oil, and fresh oregano in a wide bowl to make your dressing. Whisk the ingredients together and add salt and pepper to taste then set aside.

Take your salad bowl and mix the chickpeas, dressing, and onions together. Mix to combine and let sit to allow the onions and chickpeas marinate in the dressing for a few minutes.

Add all vegetables into the salad bowl with your chickpeas, and toss well to combine. Add the olives and fresh mint.

Serve cold or at room temperature.

Makes 2 full servings or 4 side dishes.

Warm Chickpea Salad

Chickpeas-1 15 ounce can rinsed and drained
Red seedless grapes-1 Cup, halved
Baby spinach-1 Cup
Extra virgin olive oil-2 Tbsp
Shallots-2 Tbsp, minced
Grated fresh ginger - 2 Tbsp
Lemon juice-1 Tbsp
Coarse sea salt- .25 Tsp

Using a large skillet, heat the olive oil over a medium heathen add the ginger and shallots.

Lightly saute the shallots until fragrant but not yet browned.

Carefully add the chickpeas to the skillet and stir to combine. Cook the chickpeas with the shallots for about 5 minutes until chickpeas are cooked through.

Add the lemon juice and salt over the chickpeas mixture and remove from the heat.

Toss the warm chickpeas with the spinach and grapes in a medium bowl and serve warm.

Makes 2 servings.

Broccoli Salad

Salad:

Fresh broccoli florets-5 or 6 Cups, finely chopped

Blueberries – 1.25 Cups

Dried cherries- .5 Cup

Carrots-1 Cup, shredded

Red onion- .33 Cup, finely diced

Parsley- .25 Cup, finely chopped

Cilantro- .5 Cup, finely chopped

Sliced almonds- .5 Cup, toasted

Roasted sunflower seeds- .25 Cup

Dressing:

Tahini-3 Tbsp

Warm water to thin-2 or 3 Tbsp

Fresh juiced lemon- .5

Maple syrup- .5 Tbsp

Garlic-1 Clove, minced

Salt- .25 Tsp plus additional to taste

Ground black pepper to taste

Add the broccoli, carrots, blueberries, red onion, cherries, cilantro, parsley, sunflower seeds, and toasted almonds to a large bowl then set aside.

In a small bowl, whisk together the tahini, water, lemon juice, maple syrup, garlic, salt, and pepper to make the dressing.

Drizzle the dressing over the salad and toss until well combined.

Garnish with extra toasted almonds and cilantro.

Salad will keep in an airtight container in the fridge for up to 5 days.

Makes 4 servings.

Honey Glazed Carrots

Peeled carrots-8 Medium, cut into wide match sticks
Honey- .33 Cup
Fresh parsley- .33 Cup
Butter-3 Tbsp
Turmeric-2 Tsp

Salt-1 Tsp

Ground black pepper-1 Tsp

Peeled and grated ginger-1 Inch

Squeezed and zested lemon- .5

In a skillet, melt the butter over a low to medium heat.

Add the carrots and stir to coat with the butter and add the salt.

Saute the carrots for about 2 minutes, then add the honey, turmeric, ginger, and black pepper.

Increase the heat to medium to high and continue cooking the carrots for an additional 3 minutes.

Remove the carrots from the heat and top with the lemon juice, lemon zest, and parsley.

Makes 4 servings.

Roasted Turmeric Cauliflower

Cauliflower-1 Head

Turmeric-1 Tbsp

Olive oil-1 Tbsp

A pinch of cumin

Salt and ground black pepper to taste

Preheat the oven to 400 degrees Fahrenheit.

Chop the head of cauliflower into florets and spread into a baking pan.

Add the olive oil, cumin, turmeric, and salt and mix well to coat.

Cover the baking pan with foil and roast for 35 to 40 minutes. Remove the foil and cook for an additional 15 minutes.

Makes 3-4 servings.

Golden Cauliflower Rice

Cauliflower- 4 Cups, riced

Olive oil- 1 Tbsp

Turmeric- .5 Tsp

Onion powder- .5 Tsp

Garlic powder- .5 Tsp

Ground ginger- .25 Tsp

Salt- .5 Tsp

To rice, the cauliflower, first wash it and pat it dry. Remove the outer leaves and break the head apart into 1" to 2" stemmed florets.

Add the florets into your food processor in batches and pulse 10 to 15 times until it becomes rice-sized. Remove any larger pieces left behind. You can also rice the cauliflower by hand using a large-holed grater.

Over a medium heat, warm the oil in a large skillet.

Pour the riced cauliflower and seasonings to your pan and saute the cauliflower for about 5 minutes, until it softens.

Store the cooked, riced cauliflower in a well-sealed bowl in the refrigerator for no longer than 4 days.

Makes 4 servings.

Garlic Lemon Cabbage

White cabbage-10 Cups, shredded

Lemon- .5, cut into wedges

Garlic-3 Tsp, minced

Extra virgin olive oil –2 Tsp

A pinch of crushed red pepper flakes

Fine sea salt- .5 Tsp

Warm the oil using a large skillet over a mid-level to high heated burner.

In a frying pan, add cabbage, red pepper flakes, garlic, and salt, then stir occasionally while cooking for 10 to 15 minutes until cabbage wilts down and becomes tender.

Squeeze the lemon juice over the cabbage and enjoy.

Makes 4 servings.

Lemon Garlic Broccoli

Broccoli florets- 3 Pounds

Fresh lemon juice- .25 Cup

Salt- 1 Tsp

Olive oil- .5 Cup

Garlic powder- 1 Tsp

Allow the broccoli to steam until it becomes tender then drain.

In a blender, add the oil, garlic, salt, and lemon juice and mix until it becomes creamy and smooth.

Pour the lemon sauce over the broccoli and mix until covered.

Makes 12 servings.

Garlic Spinach

Fresh spinach- 5 ounces
Garlic- 2 cloves, minced
Balsamic vinegar- 2 Dashes
Olive oil- 6 Tsp
A pinch of black pepper
A pinch of salt

Warm the garlic in the oil on a very low heat. Stir until it becomes fragrant; be sure to stir so that the garlic does not burn.

Add fresh spinach to the pan and toss in the garlic mixture to coat.

Cook the fresh spinach until it starts to wilt. Add the pepper and salt as needed and enjoy in a bowl topped with just a couple dashes of balsamic.

Makes 2 servings.

Turmeric Rice

Brown rice- 1 Cup, rinsed
Chicken broth – 1.75 Cups
Onion – 1, Diced
Cilantro–8 Ounces, chopped
Ground turmeric- 1 Tsp
Garlic- 3 Tsp, minced
Paprika - .5 Tsp
Powdered cumin- 1 Tsp
Ground black pepper- .5 Tsp
Sea salt- .5 Tsp

In a small pot, warm the oil over a mid-level heated burner. Cook the onion while stirring often for around 8 minutes.

Combine the garlic with the onion and continue cooking together for an additional60 seconds.

Next, mix the broth, rice, cumin, turmeric, pepper, salt, and paprika into the pan and mix together. Turn the cook top up to a medium/high heat to bring the water to boiling.

Once boiling, turn the heat down and allow to simmer in the saucepan while covered. Keep the rice cooking for an additional 40 minutes, then take the rice off of the burner but keep the cover on to allow it to steam for roughly 10 minutes.

Using a fork, gently stir the brown rice and toss with the cilantro.

Makes 6 servings.

Sweet Potato Fries

Sweet Potato - 1
Powdered turmeric – 1 Tsp
Coconut oil – 6 Tsp, melted
Ground cinnamon - .5 Tsp

Sea salt as needed

Turn the oven on to bake at 425 degrees Fahrenheit.

Cut the potato into long strips and pour the coconut oil and spices over them in a bowl that is about a medium size.

Toss the potatoes until well covered.

Bake the fries for around 8 to 10 minutes on a sheet pan in a single layer before flipping the sweet potatoes and allowing them to bake for 10 more minutes.

Enjoy once cooled.

Makes 1-2 servings.

Papaya Salad

Green papaya - 3 Cups, julienned
Sweet onion - .5 Cup, thinly sliced
Bean sprouts – .5 Cup
Palm sugar – 2 Tbsp, finely chopped
Lime juice – .25 Cup

Fish sauce – 2 Tbsp

Lime zest – .25 Tsp, freshly grated

Ground black pepper

Minced fresh hot or Hawaiian chiles

Whisk together the fish sauce, lime juice, sugar, chilis, and zest.

Add the papaya, bean sprouts, and onion to the vinaigrette and carefully mixuntilwell combined.

Dash with pepper as needed before serving.

Makes 6 servings.

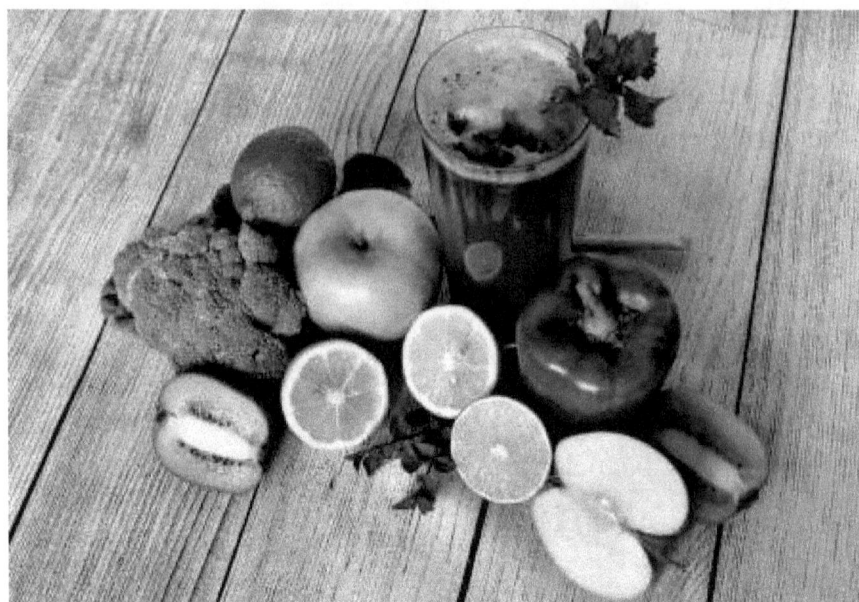

Vegetarian Dishes

Turmeric Quinoa Bowl

Yellow potatoes – 7 Small

Quinoa – .25 Cup

Chickpeas – 1 15 ounce can

Turmeric – 2 Tsp

Paprika – 1 Tsp

Kale - 2Leaves

Coconut oil – 1 Tbsp

Avocado - 1

Olive oil – .5 Tbsp

Pepper and saltas needed

Set the oven to bake at 350 degrees Fahrenheit.

Slice the yellow potatoes into strips and spread them out flat on a cooking sheet.

Lightly cover the potatoes by pouring the coconut oil and 1 teaspoon of turmeric over-top them. Add pepper and salt as needed.

Bake the potatoes for about minutes while you drain and rinse the chickpeas.

Add the chickpeas, and 1 teaspoon of paprika o a mixing bowl and coat them evenly.

Take the potatoes out of the oven and add the chickpeas to the baking sheet.

Bake the chickpeas and potatoes together for about 25 minutes to allow the potatoes to soften.

Cook the quinoa in a small saucepan. Once cooked, add in pepper, salt, and 1 teaspoon of turmeric. Toss together until well combined and allow to cool.

Wash the kale and rub the olive oil into the leaves. Divide the leaves between 4 bowls.

Carefully slice the avocado and split between the 4 bowls.

Top with the quinoa, roasted potatoes, and chickpeas then serve.

Makes 4 servings.

Lemon Soy Barley Bowl

Pearl or hulled barley – 2 Cups, cooked

Organic edam me – .75 Cups, shelled

Water – 2.25 Cups

Organic tofu (either firm or extra firm) – 1 Block of baked, savory

Ripe avocado – .5, halved and sliced thin

Lemon Tahini Dressing:

Lower sodium soy sauce – 6 Tsp

Toasted sesame oil – 3 Tsp

Dried oregano – 1.5 Tsp

Lemon – .5 Tsp, finely grated

Juice of .5 of a lemon

Bring the barley and water to boiling in a medium saucepan.

Once boiling, reduce the heat down to low so that the barley can simmer for about 40 to 50 minutes. It is done once all of the liquid has been absorbed.

Take the barley off of the burner so that it may cool just slightly.

Whisk the sesame oil, oregano, soy sauce, lemon zest, and lemon juice in a large bowl until they have combined well.

Pour or scoop the cooled barley into the large bowl and stir to cover with the soy mix.

Then, drop the edam me and arugula into the barley mix and continue to gently toss until combined.

Cut the tofu into ¾ inch cubes.

Divide the barley mixture between 4 bowls and serve topped with avocado slices and tofu.

Makes 4 servings.

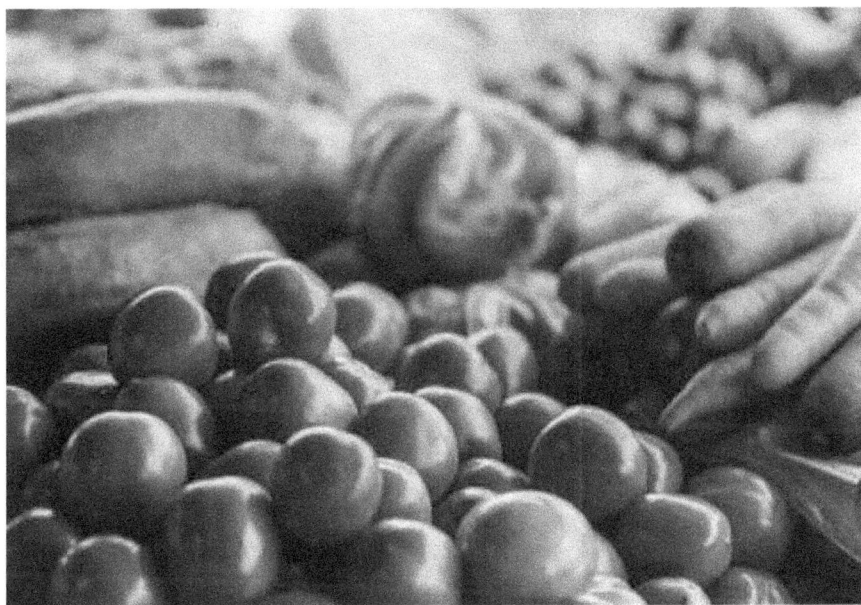

Avocado Egg Salad Sandwiches

Ripe avocado – .5

Avocado oil – 1 Tsp

Organic hard-boiled eggs – 3 Chopped

Lemon juice – 1.5 Tsp

Celery – .25 Cup, finely chopped

Fresh chives – 3 Tsp, chopped

Salt – .25 Tsp

Black pepper – .125 Tsp

Whole wheat sandwich bread – 4 Slices

Lettuce – 2 Leaves

In a medium bowl, scoop the flesh of the half avocado, add the lemon juice, and avocado oil. Mash until almost smooth.

To the mixture of avocado, add the celery, pepper, salt, eggs, and chives then stir until well combined.

Spread the mixture onto 2 pieces of toast, then add a lettuce leaf and another piece of toast to make 2 sandwiches.

Makes 2 servings.

Chickpea Lettuce Wraps

Chickpea filling:
Chickpeas – 1 Can, drained and rinsed
Garlic - 1Clove, chopped
Spring onion – 1 Chopped
Turmeric – 1 Tsp
Sesame seeds – 3 Tsp
Cumin – 1 Tsp
Flax seeds – 3 Tsp
Ground chili pepper – 1 Tsp
Olive oil – 1 Tbsp

Mint - 6Leaves

Salad:
Avocado - 1
Garlic – 1 Clove, chopped
Tomatoes – 2 Diced
Pointed green pepper – 1 Chopped
Spring onion – 1 Chopped
Basil leaves - 12
Walnuts – 2 Tbsp, crushed
Lime juice – 1 Tsp
Romaine lettuce – 6 Leaves, washed

Heat chickpeas over a mid-level to high heated burner in a frying pan with about a ¼ cup of water. Add turmeric and chili powder and stir until the chickpeas are well coated. Cook about 2 to 3 minutes.

Once all water is almost gone, add the remaining filling ingredients. Stir together for approximately60 seconds, then cover and turn them off on the cook top.

Smash together the avocado with half of the diced tomatoes. Pour in the lime juice and minced garlic, stir together until the mixture is well combined, and lumps have been removed.

Add in the remaining salad ingredients along with some salt to taste. Stir to combine.

Top salad mixture with crushed walnuts.

Add 2 tbsp of the chickpea filling to the middle of the lettuce leaves and top with 2 tablespoons of the salad.

Enjoy!

Makes 6 servings.

Chickpea Cakes

Onion – 1 Small

Chickpeas – 1 Can, rinsed and drained

Garlic – 2 Cloves

Fresh parsley – .25 Cup, chopped

Sea salt – 1.5 Tsp

Powdered turmeric – 1 Tsp

Potato starch – 6 Tsp

Cayenne pepper – .75 Tsp

Chickpea flour – 2 Tbsp plus 3 extra tablespoons for coating

Grape seed oil

Fresh ground black pepper

Drizzle a little grape seed oil into a large cast-iron pan and saute the garlic and onion until just slightly golden brown. Take off the burner and set aside to cool.

Mix the chickpeas using a blending appliance. Once they become a smooth, thick consistency, turn the blender off and use a small spatula or spoon to be sure none of the chickpeas are stuck to the sides, and all have been ground.

To the blender add, the garlic, onion, pepper, salt, cayenne pepper, and turmeric to the chickpea mix and blend until well mixed.

Turn the blender off again and use a spoon to manually mix in the chopped parsley.

Add 3 tablespoons of chickpea flour to a large plate.

Scoop out some of the chickpea mixture using a spoon and form into a golf ball-sized ball. Press the ball gently to make flatten into a patty-like shape.

Drop the patty into the chickpea flour to give it a light even coat on both sides.

Repeat forming and coating the patties until all of the chickpea mixture is gone.

Put the cast iron pan back onto the cook top and heat to medium. Pour in just a small amount of additional oil and cook the patties for about 2 or 3 minutes per side until they are brown.

Serve over a salad.

Makes 4 servings.

Avocado Chickpea Sandwich

Chickpeas – 1 15 ounce can drained and rinsed
Lemon juice – 2 Tsp
Ripe avocado – 1 Large
Dried cranberries – .25 Cup
Salt and pepper to taste

Toppings:
Arugula

Red onion

4 Slices of whole grain bread is optional. Avocado and chickpea can be enjoyed over a salad.

In a medium-sized bowl, mash the chickpeas using a fork.

Combine the avocado with the chickpeas and continue to mash with fork until somewhat smooth and well combined.

Add the lemon juice and dried cranberries to the avocado mix, stir until well combined and sprinkle with additional salt and pepper as needed.

Toast bread and spread the mixture over 2 pieces of toast.

Top with arugula, red onion, and another slice of toast. Enjoy!

Avocado mixture can be Store the avocado mixture for up to 2 days in the refrigerator.

Makes 2 servings.

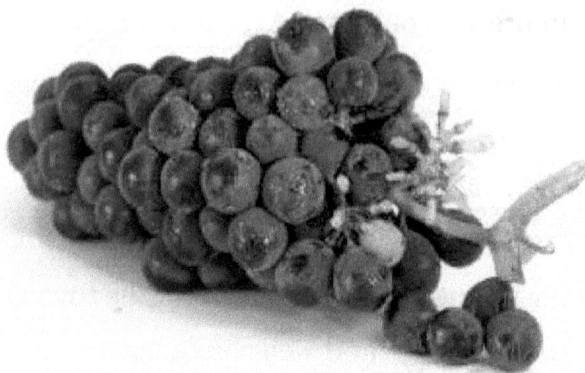

Red Lentil Pasta

Red lentil pasta – 1 8ounce box

Extra virgin olive oil – .25 Cup

Garlic - 6 cloves, minced

Sweet onion – 1 Chopped

Dried oregano – 1 Tbsp

Dried basil – 3 Tsp

Ground turmeric – 2 Tsp

Apple cider vinegar – 3 Tsp

Fire-roasted tomatoes – 1 28 ounce can

Baby spinach – 2 Large handfuls

½ Cup of chopped, Sun-dried tomatoes – .5 Cup, chopped and oil drained

Pepper and salt as needed

Grated parmesan

Toasted pine nuts or seeds

Over a medium heat, use a pot to warm the oil.

Once the olive oil has been heated, saute the onion until just softened, and it is beginning to carmelize. (about 5 to 10 minutes)

To the pot, add the oregano, basil, pepper, garlic, salt, and turmeric, then cook for about 1 minute to allow flavors to combine.

Slowly, add the tomatoes and juice from the can into the pot.

Using a potato masher, crush the tomatoes in the pot.

Pour in the vinegar and sun-dried tomatoes, and while occasionally stirring, allow to simmer until sauce reduces slightly about 12 to 15 minutes.

Put the greens in with the tomatoes then allow to simmer for another few minutes.

Bring salted water to boiling in another pot large enough for the pasta.

Pour in the noodles, boil while stirring occasionally until it reaches your desired doneness then drain.

Divide between 6 bowls and mix in the sauce. Add cheese, nuts, and seeds if you'd like.

Makes 6 servings.

Cauliflower Chickpea Salad

Chickpeas – 1 cup rinsed and drained
Red tipped leaf lettuce – 2 Cups, torn
Cauliflower florets – 1.5 Cups
Red onion - .25 Cup, sliced thin
Carrots - .75 Cup, cut into .5" slices
Plain fat-free yogurt - .25 Cup
Powdered curry – 3 Tsp
Olive oil – 3 Tsp
Salt - .25 Tsp

Lime juice – 1 Tbsp

Ground black pepper - .5 Tsp

Ground ginger - .25 Tsp

½ Teaspoon of minced jalapeno pepper

Set the oven to bake at 450 degrees Fahrenheit.

Stir together the salt, olive oil, and curry powder in a medium bowl, then add in the chickpeas, cauliflower, and carrots. Mix to fully coat.

Spread the cauliflower, carrots, and chickpeas onto a sheet pan and cook in the oven for 20-25 minutes. Stir once about halfway through. Veggies are done once softened. Take them out of the oven and allow to cool.

To make your dressing, stir together the yogurt, lime juice, jalapeno pepper, and ginger in a small bowl. Thin with a little water if you prefer it to be a bit thinner.

Using a salad bowl, mix the lettuce, veggies, onion, and parsley. Pour in the dressing and toss to coat.

Makes 2 servings.

Stuffed Sweet Potato

Sweet potato – 1 Large
Black beans – 1 Cup, drained and rinsed
Hummus - .25 Cup
Kale - .75 Cup, chopped
Water – 2 Tbsp

Poke the sweet potato a few times with a fork and microwave on high for about 7 to 10 minutes until cooked through.

Wash the kale and drain. Cook the kale, covered, over a mid-level heat. Stir the kale a couple of times until wilted.

Add beans and 1 to 2 tablespoons of water if the saucepan is dry.

Continue to cook the beans and kale uncovered for about 1 to 2 minutes until the mixture is hot, stirring occasionally.

Split the sweet potato open lengthwise along the top and stuff with the beans and kale.

Mix together the hummus and 2 tablespoons of water in a small dish until desired consistency and then drizzle over the stuffed potato.

Makes 1 serving.

Vegetable Stir Fry

Fresh broccoli florets – 4 Cups

Fresh ginger - .25 Cup, minced

Garlic – 12 cloves, minced

Green onions – 1 Bunch, sliced

Water chestnuts – 1 Cup, chopped

Mushrooms – 1 Cup, chopped

Sugar snap peas – 1 Cup

Red bell pepper – 1 Sliced

Sesame oil – 1 Tbsp

Brown rice for serving if desired

Stir Fry Sauce:

1Reduced sodium soy sauce - .33 Cup plus 2 Tbsp

Sesame oil - .25 Cup

Cornstarch – 1 Tbsp

Heat sesame oil over a mid-level to high heated burner.

Pour the bell pepper, water chestnuts, sugar snap peas, mushrooms, onion, garlic, broccoli, and ginger into the oil and cook for 20 to 25 minutes stirring often to keep from burning. To make the stir fry sauce, add the 3 ingredients to a mason jar, screw the lid on, and shake to combine. Sauce with thicken as it cooks.

Once the vegetables are cooked but not too soft and the liquid evaporates from the pan add in the stir fry sauce and continue to cook for another 3 to 5 minutes. Continue to stir often and make sure the sauce fully coats all of the vegetables.

Stir fry can be enjoyed as is or served over brown rice.

Makes 6 servings.

Crockpot Chili

Tomatoes – 3 Cups, diced
Kidney beans – 3 Cups, cooked
Water - .5 Cup
Mushrooms – 8 Ounces, sliced
Onion– 1 Diced
Green bell pepper – 1 Chopped

Garlic cloves – 2, Minced

Fresh or frozen corn kernels (not canned) – 1 Cup

Zucchini – 1 Diced

Chili powder – 6 Tsp

Cumin – 2 Tsp

Oregano - .5 Tsp

Cayenne pepper to taste

Add all items to your crockpot and manually mix until fully combined.

Heat, covered, for 7 hours on a low setting.

Makes 4 servings.

Butternut Squash Soup

Butternut squash – 2 Peeled and cubed

Apple – 1 Large, peeled and chopped

Vegetable broth – 1.25 Cups

Onion - .5 Cup, chopped

Heavy whipping cream - .5 Cup

Salt – 1 Tsp

Cayenne pepper - .125 tsp

Spray your slow cooking crock with nonstick cooking spray and add all ingredients except for the heavy whipping cream. Mix together.

Heat, covered in your cooker for 4-5 hours on the high setting.

Pour half of the squash soup into a blending appliance and allow it to cool, then cover and mix until well combined and lumps are removed.

Transfer the soup to a large dish then repeat to blend the remaining half of the squash mixture.

Pour all of the blended soup back to the crock of your slow cooker and manually mix the whipping cream in.

Replace the cover on your slow cooker and allow to heat for another few minutes so that the soup is fully heated and combined.

Makes 6 servings.

Roasted Squash Penne

Squash:

Delicata squash – 2 Medium, scrubbed and rinsed

Olive oil – 2 Tbsp

Sea salt as needed

Ground black pepper as needed

Walnut Pesto:

Fresh parsley – 1 Cup

Walnut halves - .75 Cups, toasted

Garlic - 3Cloves

Sage – 6 Large leaves

Roasted walnut oil - .5 Cup

Salt as needed

Ground black pepper as needed

Pasta:

Whole wheat penne – 1 Pound, uncooked

Parmesan - .5 Cup, grated

Extra virgin olive oil - .25 Cup

Fresh sage leaves for frying

Preheat oven to 425 degrees Fahrenheit.

Cover a sheet pan with a silicone pad and put to the side until needed.

Bring salted water to a boil for the pasta.

Trim the ends of the squash and slice them in half lengthwise.

Use a spoon to scoop the seeds out of the squash.

Cut each half of the squash into ½", half-moon slices and place onto the lined baking sheet.

Pour some oil over the squash and season with some pepper and salt. Spread evenly in the pan, so they are not touching.

Put the squash into the oven to roast for 10 to 15 minutes, then take the squash out of oven to flip. Continue to roast for an additional 10 to 12 minutes; the squash should be tender.

While the squash is roasting, combine the walnuts, parsley, garlic, and sage leaves and pulse in your food processor until coarsely chopped. Pour in the walnut oil and continue to pulse, it should be almost smooth. Add pepper and salt and move pesto to a bowl.

Cover a small plate with paper towels and heat a small amount of olive oil over a mid-level to high heated burner. Saute the sage leaves a few at a time until crisp then transfer to the covered plate. Lightly salt and put to the side.

Pour the pasta into the pot of boiling water and boil until desired doneness. Set aside 8 ounces of the water the pasta was cooked in, then remove the remaining water from the pasta. Pour a small amount of olive oil into the pasta and mix in until combined well and coated. Add to the pasta, the grated parmesan cheese, and pesto. Lightly mix until the sauce is evenly covering the pasta, adding some of the pasta water that had been set aside as needed for a creamier sauce.

Serve the pasta topped with the squash pieces and garnish with the fried sage leaves.

Makes 4-6 servings.

Curried Potato with Poached Egg

Russet potatoes - 2

Tomato sauce – 15 Ounce can

Organic eggs – 4 Large

Fresh ginger – 1 Inch

Olive oil – 3 Tsp

Garlic cloves – 2

Curry powder – 2 Tbsp

Fresh cilantro - .5 Bunch, chopped

Rinse the potatoes and dice into cubes about ¾" in size. Cover the potatoes with water in a large pot.

Put a cover on the pot and bring water to a boil over high heat. Boil the potatoes until easily pierced with a fork then drain.

Peel the ginger with a vegetable peeler and use a small holed grater to grate about 1" of ginger then mince the garlic.

Sauté on a medium/low heat, garlic, ginger, and olive oil in a large skillet for 1 to 2 minutes before adding the curry and continuing to saute for about another minute or so.

Turn the heat up slightly and carefully pour in the tomato sauce. Cook while stirring until heated. Then taste and add additional seasoning if needed.

Stir the potatoes into the skillet until well coated.

Create 4 small dips in the potato mixture and crack 1 egg into each dip. Put a lid on the skillet and allow it to simmer in the sauce until eggs are cooked to your liking, about 6 to 10 minutes.

Top with fresh cilantro.

Makes 4 servings.

Crunchy Cinnamon Granola

Unsweetened shredded coconut - .25 Cup
Old-fashioned rolled oats – 2 Cups
Raisins - .25 Cup
Dried apricots - .25 Cup, chopped
Walnuts - .25 Cup, chopped
Honey - .25 Cup
Dried cranberries - .25 Cup
Pumpkin seeds – 2 Tbsp
Unsalted butter – 4 tbsp, melted
Ground cloves - .25 Tsp
Powdered cinnamon - .5 Tsp
Powdered nutmeg - .25 Tsp

Turn your oven on to bake at 300 degrees Fahrenheit.

Cover a sheet pan with a silicone pad and put aside.

Combine the oats, pumpkin seeds, shredded coconut, walnuts, and spices together then put to the side until needed.

Pour the melted butter and honey together in a separate bowl then stir until fully mixed. Drizzle the honey over your oat mixture.

Scoop out the honey-covered oats and spread them evenly on your baking sheet. Allow the mixture to cook in the oven for around half an hour. Once it is beginning to brown, take the mixture out and allow it to cool.

Once the granola has cooled, break it up and stir in the remaining ingredients.

The granola can be stored at room temperature in an airtight container.

Makes 3.5 cups.

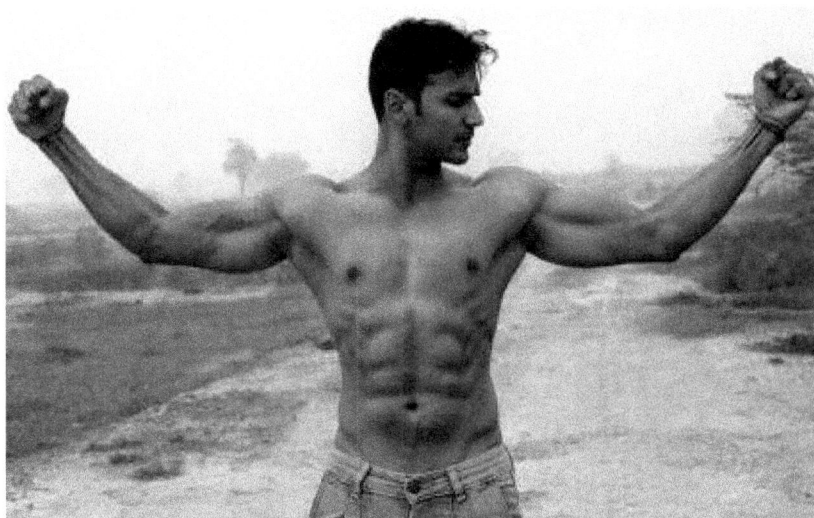

Fish and Seafood Dishes

<u>Salmon Bowl</u>

Cauliflower rice – 1 Cup

Purple cabbage - .25 Cup, shredded

Edam me - .33 Cup, shelled

Mixed greens such as kale and collard greens – 2 Cups, chopped

Fresh basil – 2 Tbsp

Hemp seeds – 2 Tsp

Fresh mint – 2 Tbsp

Walnuts - .25 Cup, chopped

Salmon – 2, 5 Ounce skin on fillets

Sunflower sprouts for garnish

Miso Ginger Dressing:

Garlic – 1 Clove, minced

Tahini – 3 Tbsp

White miso – 1 Tbsp

Rice vinegar – 3 Tbsp

Freshly grated ginger – 1 Tbsp

Water to thin as needed

Blend together all dressing ingredients until smooth. Use water to thin as needed and transfer the dressing to a jar or bottle.

Mix together in a large bowl, the cauliflower rice, purple cabbage, edam me, fresh herbs, and a few tablespoons of the dressing. Put to the side to let the flavors mix.

Spray a frying pan with avocado oil or olive oil. Add in the mixed greens, 1 tablespoon of dressing and 2 tablespoons of water.

Cook the greens are stirring frequently until just beginning to wilt but still bright in color.

Divide the greens between 2 bowls.

Put the pan back onto the heated burner and respray with oil if needed.

Fry the fillets skin side up in a frying pan for about 4 to 5 minutes or until you can see from the side that it is cooked about ¾ of the way through.

Flip each fillet and fry for 2 additional minutes. Take the frying pan off of the burner.

Scoop half of the"rice" into one bowl and the remaining half in the other. Serve it over the greens.

Peel the skin off of the salmon and stack a fillet over each rice bowl.

Sprinkle the bowls with chopped walnuts, sunflower sprouts, and hemp seeds.

Drizzle with dressing and enjoy.

Makes 2 servings.

Smoked Salmon Tartine

Potato Tartine:
Clarified butter – 2 Tbsp
1 Large Russet potato – 1 Large, peeled and grated
Black pepper and saltas needed

Toppings:

Soft goat cheese – 4 Ounces at room temperature
Chives – 1.5 Tbsp

Red onion – 2 Tbsp, finely diced

Capers – 2 Tbsp, drained

Garlic - .5Clove, minced

Hard-boiled egg - .5Finely chopped

Smoked salmon, thinly sliced

Zest of half a lemon

Finely minced chives for garnish

Mix together the garlic, lemon zest, and goat cheese. Add salt and black pepper, then add the chives to the mix and set aside.

Add some salt to the hard-boiled egg and red onion.

Working quickly, use a large hole grater, grate the potato into a larger sized bowl.

Squeeze the potato over the sink or a bowl to drain the excess liquid.

Add a generous amount of pepper and salt to the potatoes.

Over a medium/high heat, warm the clarified butter in a nonstick skillet.

Once the butter has heated, shape the grated potatoes into a large circle in the skillet using a spatula.

Using the spatula once again, press the potatoes down into the hot pan. Pan-fry the potatoes, covered for about 8 minutes until browned.

Carefully flip it over and allow the other side to brown as well for about 8 more minutes.

Once potatoes are crispy and golden brown, take them out of the pan and place them on a cooling rack until room temperature.

Add the goat cheese on top of the cooled potato cake.

Lay the smoked salmon over the cheese mixture and top with the hard-boiled egg, capers, and red onion.

If desired, top with chives to garnish and serve cut into wedges.

Makes 1-2 servings.

Quinoa Shrimp Avocado Bowl

Crispy Kale:

Olive oil – 2 Tbsp

Kale – 1 Bunch, roughly torn

Black pepper and salt to taste

Quinoa:

Olive oil – 2 Tbsp

Quinoa – 1.25 Cups

Chicken broth – 2 Cups

Salt and pepper

Spicy Shrimp and Toppings:

Shrimp – 1 Pound, deveined and peeled

Watermelon radishes – 2 Thinly sliced

Ripe avocados – 2 Peeled, pitted and sliced

Extra virgin olive oil – 3 Tsp

Powdered cumin – 1 Tsp

Hot sauce – 2 Tbsp

Powdered coriander - .75 Tsp

Salt and pepper

Turn the oven on to bake at 400 degrees Fahrenheit

Cover a sheet pan using a silicone pad.

Mix together the kale and olive oil. Season with pepper and salt if desired.

Arrange the kale on a sheet pan without overlapping and then bake until crisp. (about 15 minutes)

While the kale is in oven, over medium heat, warm the oil in a medium-sized pot.

Pour the quinoa into the pot and toast for about 1 minute in the olive oil while constantly stirring.

Carefully pourin the broth in the pot over the quinoa and let it simmer.

Continue to simmer the quinoa until there is no longer any liquid and it has softened.

Season with some pepper and a little salt and put the quinoa to the side for now.

Heat the oil on a mid-level to high setting on your cook top.

In a medium-sized bowl, toss the shrimp with the cumin, coriander, and hot sauce.

Sprinkle pepper and salt over the shrimp and saute for about 4 to 5 minutes in the frying pan until fully cooked.

Split the quinoa between 4 bowls and top each with the kale and shrimp.

Add the sliced avocado and watermelon radishes to the top of each bowl and serve immediately.

Makes 4 servings.

Salmon Taco Wrap

Fresh Salmon - 2Fillets
Coleslaw mix or shredded cabbage – 2 or 3 Cups
Butter lettuce – 1 Head
Fresh cilantro - .25 Cup
Grilled fish seasoning – 1.5 Tbsp
Juiced lime - 1
Salt to taste
Avocado oil

Mayo:

Avocado oil – 1 Cup

Organic egg – 1 Large

Juiced lemon – 1 Tsp

Salt - .25 Tsp

Dijon mustard - .5 Tsp

Avocado Sauce:

Avocado - .5, Pitted

Fresh cilantro - .5 Cup

Jalapeno - .5 Seeded

Water - .25 Cup

Garlic – 1 Clove

Salt - .5 Tsp

First, make the mayo by pouring all ingredients into a glass jar and inserting an immersion blender. Bring blender all the way down to the bottom of the jar, making sure you have taken the egg with it and blend at the bottom until the mixture becomes a white and creamy then slower move blender back up through the jar to ensure all is blended together.

Next, prepare the avocado sauce by adding all of the ingredients plus ½ of a cup of the mayo to a blender and combining until smooth. Add a little water and continue to blend if the sauce needs to be thinned out.

Season the salmon fillets with the grilled fish seasoning and lightly pat them to get the seasoning to stick well then drizzle with some Avocado oil.

Heat your grill to a mid-level heat, then cook the salmon for around 5 to 8 minutes, flipping once. Do not overcook as they will dry out. Take the salmon off the grill and put it to the side to allow it to cool.

In a small bowl, combine slaw with chopped cilantro and lime juice. Add salt if desired.

Rinse the lettuce leaves and pat dry using a paper towel. Select the best cup-shaped leaves to use for the taco wraps.

Once the salmon has cooled, break it apart and place the pieces into the lettuce wraps and lightly cover each with the slaw mixture.

Top the tacos with avocado sauce.

Makes 4-6 servings.

Seafood Chowder

Salmon - .33 Pound of skinless fillet

Cod - .33 Pound of skinless fillet

Bone broth – 1 Qt

Full fat coconut cream - .5 Cup

White sweet potato – 1 Small, peeled and diced

Fennel bulb – 1 Small, finely chopped

Carrots – 3 Peeled and diced

Celery ribs – 3 Finely chopped

Thyme – 1.5 Tbsp, minced

Olive oil – 3 Tbsp

Bay leaf - 1

Fine sea salt to taste

Saute the celery, carrots, sweet potato, fennel, thyme, and bay leaf for about 10 minutes in heated olive oil in a stockpot on a mid-level heated burner. Stir frequently. Don't allow the vegetables to brown or stick; add more oil if needed.

Carefully pour in the broth and raise the heat until it boils. Add the fish to the boiling pot and turn the burner down to mid-level. Continue cooking for an additional 8-10 minutes.

Once the vegetables have become soft, and the fish is thoroughly done, take out and discard the bay leaf and put the fish on a plate using a slotted spoon. Break the fish into smaller pieces watching for any bones that may have been left.

Stir the pieces of fish after placing them back into the pot with the coconut cream. Sprinkle some salt into the chowder if desired.

Right before serving, garnish with fresh thyme.

Makes 4 servings.

Shrimp Fajitas

Yellow bell pepper – 1 thinly sliced
Shrimp – 1.5 Pounds raw, deveined and peeled
Red bell pepper – 1,Cut into thin slices
Red onion – 1 small, cut into thin slices
Orange bell pepper – 1, Cut into thin slices
Olive oil – .5 Tbsp
Garlic Powder - .5 Tsp
Chili powder – .5 Tbsp
Salt – 1 Tsp
Ground cumin - .5 Tsp

Paprika - .5 Tsp

Onion powder - .5 Tsp

Lime

Warmed tortillas

Turn the oven on to bake at 450 degrees Fahrenheit.

Toss together the bell peppers, olive oil, shrimp, onions, pepper, salt, and spices. Mix well.

Use non-stick cooking spray to spray a sheet pan and lay the mixture out so that none the ingredients are covering the others.

Roast for about 8 minutes then switch a low broil for another 2 minutes to ensure shrimp is done.

Take the fajita mix out of the oven and squeeze fresh lime juice over it. Top with fresh cilantro and serve in tortillas.

Makes 4 servings.

Mediterranean Cod

Cod – 1 Pound cut into 4 portions

Diced tomatoes – 1 14.5 ounce can

Kale – 2 Cups, shredded

Fennel – 2 Cups, sliced

Fresh diced tomatoes – 1 Cup

Black olives – 1 Cup

Water - .5 Cup

Onion – 1 Small, sliced

Olive oil – 2 Tbsp

Garlic – 3 Large cloves, chopped

Fresh oregano – 2 Tsp

Salt - .125 Tsp

Fennel seeds - .25 Tsp

Ground black pepper - .25 Tsp

Orange zest – 1 Tsp

A pinch of crushed red pepper

Garnish:

Fresh oregano, fennel fronds, olive oil, orange zest, etc.

Heat the oil on a mid-level to high burner. Cook the fennel, garlic, and onion for 8 minutes and sprinkle with pepper and salt to taste. Add the water, tomatoes, and kale. Stir until well combined, and for about 10 to 12 minutes, allow it to simmer.

To the skillet, toss in the crushed red pepper, oregano, and olives.

Season the fish with orange zest, pepper, fennel seeds, and salt.

Put the fish into trepan with the tomato and kale mix and cover.

Allow the fish to cook through for about 10 minutes then take the skillet off of the burner.

Garnish the mixture and serve.

Makes 4 servings.

Shrimp and Cauliflower Grits

Shrimp:
Shrimp – 1 Pound, large
No salt Cajun seasoning – 2.5 Tbsp
Butter or ghee – 2 Tbsp
Salt

Cauliflower Grits:
Frozen cauliflower – 1 12 ounce bag
Garlic – 1 Large clove, chopped

Butter – 2 tbsp

Salt as needed

Bring a couple inches of water to a rolling boil. Using a steamer basket, place the cauliflower and chopped garlic over the boing water, steam while covered until the cauliflower has softened.

Once the cauliflower is ready, pulse it in a blender or food processor with butter until it reaches a grit like consistency. Add salt and just a little of the steaming water and pulse again until it reaches the desired consistency.

Pat the shrimp dry and season well with Cajun seasoning and salt.

Melt the butter over a mid-level to high burner. Sauté the seasoned shrimp in the hot skillet for 1 to 2 minutes until shrimp is just turning pink. Then remove from skillet.

Serve cauliflower grits in your bowls and lay the shrimp on top. Pour the butter and Cajun sauce from the skillet over the bowls and serve.

Makes 2 servings.

Salmon Cakes

Salmon – 5 Ounces, cooked, peeled and finely diced
Organic eggs – 2 Large
Coconut flour – 3 or 4 Tbsp
Sweet potato - .33 Cup, mashed
Garlic - .5 Tsp, minced
Ground black pepper - .25 Tsp
Paprika - .25 Tsp
Rosemary – 1 Sprig
Sea salt - .25 Tsp
Butter – 1 Tbsp
Curry powder - .25 Tsp

Mash the salmon and mix it in a bowl with the sweet potato.

Add the flour to the bowl slowly, then stir in the seasoning and herbs until combined well.

Add the eggs to your salmon and sweet potato and combine well. After the batter becomes thick enough, form 8 small patties or 5 to 6 larger patties.

Warm the oil on a mid-level to high burner on your cook top. Cook the patties in batches in the hot butter on each side for about 3 to 4 minutes until the salmon is thoroughly cooked.

Garnish the patties with ground black pepper, rosemary or garlic.

Serve with steamed veggies, or alone as an appetizer.

Makes 3-4 servings.

Salmon Blueberry Salad

Salad:
Smoked salmon – 6 Ounces, thinly sliced
Baby spinach – 2 Cups
Fresh blueberries - .5 Cup
Watercress – 2 Cups
Raw unsalted walnut pieces – .25 Cup
Red onion – 2.5 Tbsp, minced
Fresh basil – 1 Tbsp
Ripe avocado - .5 Small, diced
Fresh mint – 1 Tbsp, thinly sliced

Garnish with sunflower, sprouts, peas, etc.

Ginger Citrus Vinaigrette:
Orange juice - .33 Cup, freshly squeezed
Apple cider vinegar – 6 Tsp
Extra virgin olive oil - .5 Cup
Dijon mustard – 2 Tsp
Raw honey – 2 Tsp
Fresh ginger – 1 Tsp, finely grated
Ground black pepper and sea salt

In a glass jar, add all vinaigrette items, cover, and shake until well combined.
Add some pepper and salt then set aside.

Wash the spinach and trim if needed. Use a paper towel to dry it and toss it into a large bowl along with blueberries, herbs, and walnuts.

Add some vinaigrette to the salad and mix until well covered.

Gently mix in the avocado and divide the salad between 2 bowls.

Split the salmon between the bowls and add the sprouts to garnish.

Serve with additional dressing if preferred.

Makes 2 servings.

Cod with Roasted Tomatoes

Cod – 4 Fresh 4ounce skinless fillets

Cherry tomatoes – 3 Cups

Fresh oregano – 2 Tsp, chopped

Fresh thyme – 1 Tsp, chopped

Capers – 2 Tsp

Powdered garlic - .25 Tsp

Paprika - .25 Tsp

Salt - .5 Tsp

Garlic – 2 cloves, sliced

Black pepper - .25 Tsp

Black olives – 2 Tbsp, pitted and sliced

Olive oil – 1 Tbsp

Fresh oregano

Turn oven on to bake at 450 degrees Fahrenheit.

Rinse off the fish and then use paper towels to dry it.

Stir together, oregano, thyme, salt, paprika, powdered garlic, and pepper. Using half of the mixture season both sides of the fillets.

Use aluminum foil to cover a sheet pan and then spray the foil with a non-stick spray.

Lay the fish out on one half of the foil and then arrange the garlic slices and tomatoes on the other half.

Combine the olive oil with the remaining oregano mixture and drizzle onto the tomatoes. Mix until well coated.

Bake for 8 to 12 minutes, stirring the tomato mixture once. Test fish for doneness by using a fork to see if it flakes easily.

Remove from oven and stir capers and olives into the tomato mix.

Garnish with fresh oregano and enjoy.

Makes 4 servings.

Lemon Salmon with Zucchini

Salmon:

Salmon–4 5 ounce fillets

Garlic – 2 cloves, minced

Dried dill - .5 Tsp

Brown sugar – 2 Tbsp, packed

Dried oregano - .5 Tsp

Lemon juice – 2 Tbsp, fresh squeezed

Parsley – 6 Tsp, fresh chopped

Dijon mustard – 1 Tbsp

Dried rosemary - .25 Tsp

Dried thyme - .25 Tsp

Ground black pepper and salt as needed

Zucchini – 4 Chopped

Olive oil – 2 Tbsp

Salt and pepper as needed

Turn oven on to bake at 400 degrees Fahrenheit and oil a baking pan, lightly.

Mix the Dijon, brown sugar, dill, lemon juice, thyme, rosemary, garlic, and oregano. Add pepper and salt and set aside.

Lay the zucchini out on a sheet pan in one even layer, then season with the pepper and salt and pour the oil over the top. Lay the salmon onto the sheet and brush the fillet with the herb mix.

Cook in the oven for around 16 to 18 minutes until the fish flakes easily.

Serve garnished with parsley.

Makes 4 servings.

Crab Fried "Rice"

King crab legs – 1 Pound, frozen

Cauliflower – 24 Ounces, riced

Organic eggs – 2 Large, beaten

Onion - .5 Finely diced

Garlic – 2 cloves, minced

Sesame oil – 3 Tsp

Low sodium soy sauce – .125Cup

Scallions – 5 Diced with whites and greens separated

A pinch of salt

Nonstick cooking spray

Riced cauliflower can be purchased frozen or to make it yourself, place florets into a blending appliance or processor in small batches and pulse repeatedly until it is the desired size. It can also be grated using a large whole grater for a similar texture.

Boil a couple of inches of water in a pot large enough for your crab legs. Carefully drop the crab legs to the pot of boiling water and cook with the cover on for roughly 10 minutes. Once the crab is fully cooked, take it off of the burner. Take the meat out of the shell and flake it lightly.

Use the non-stick spray on your wok or a deep pan for frying and warm on a mid-level heat. Sprinkle some salt on the eggs and cook while stirring occasionally until they have set. Take the eggs out and put to the side.

Pour the sesame oil into the panthen turn the burner down to a low. Saute the scallion whites, onion, and garlic for around 3 to 4 minutes, stirring frequently until they soften.

Once again, turn up the burner to a mid-level/high heat, then pour the soy and riced cauliflower into the pan. Mix with the garlic and onions, then cook, covered, foran additional 5 to 6 minutes while stirring often. "Rice" is ready when it starts to crisp a little on the inside but is still soft on the inside.

Return the crab and egg to the pan, mix well and take the pan off of the burner. Mix in the green scallions and serve.

Makes 4 servings.

Salmon with Zoodles

Wild salmon – 1 Pound
Zucchini noodles – 3 Cups
Olives - .75 Cup
Grape tomatoes - .75 Cup
Garlic – 4 cloves, crushed
Red onion – 1 Small, sliced
Sea salt - .25 Tsp
Olive oil – 6 Tsp
Za'atar – 1 Tsp
        (can be substituted with a little dried thyme and oregano)
Fresh lemon wedges
Black pepper as needed

Turn the oven on to bake at 400 degrees Fahrenheit.

Drizzle about 1 teaspoon of oil over the salmon then season using 1 clove of garlic, salt, and za'atar. Za'atar can be found in middle eastern markets and specialty stores but dried thyme and oregano work just as well.

Place fish in the center of a sheet pan.

Mix the zucchini noodles, remaining garlic, olives, tomato, onion, pepper, and oil. Lay the zoodles mix onto the baking sheet and layout, taking care not to overlap or cover the fish.

Oven roast for about 10 minutes then take the fish out of the oven served with a lemon wedge and a little salt

Makes 3 servings.

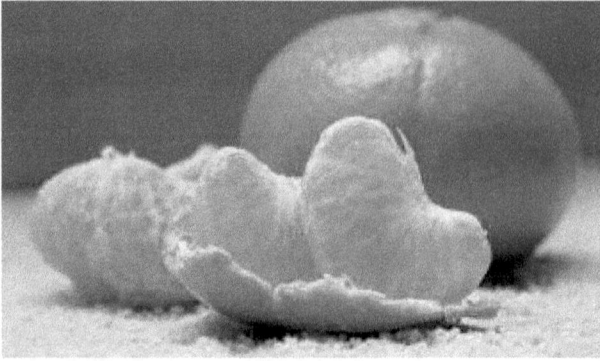

Broiled Bass and Tomatoes

Striped bass – 4 6 ounce fillets

Heirloom tomatoes – 3 Medium, diced

Mixed olives - .33 Cup, pitted and chopped

Olive oil – 6 Tsp

Dijon mustard – 3 Tsp

White wine vinegar – 3 Tsp

Capers – 3 Tsp

Cloves of garlic– 1, minced

Optional Herbs de Provence

A mix of chopped herbs such as thyme, parsley, chives, etc.

Sea Salt as needed

Clean the fish under cold water and then dry the fish fillet using a paper towel. Spread the fillets out onto a sheet pan and season with some salt and Herbs de Provence.

Spread Dijon mustard over the top of the bass.

Stir together the tomatoes, olives, capers, garlic, vinegar, olive oil, and about ½ a teaspoon of sea salt until combined well, then layout over the fish.

Broil on low for about 5 minutes, keeping an eye on it as it can burn quickly. Then rotate the pan and broil for 5 minutes longer or until tomatoes are starting to caramelize and fish is cooked.

Top with the herbs and serve with a side salad.

Makes 4 servings.

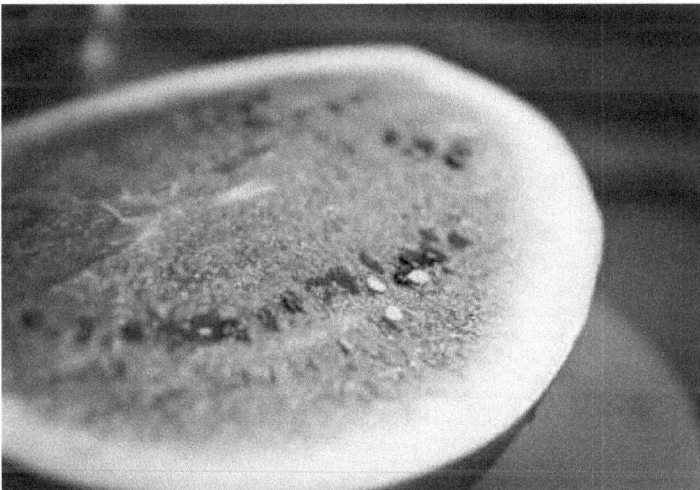

Meat and Poultry Dishes

<u>Chicken Enchilada Bowl</u>

Cilantro Lime Cauliflower Rice:

Chili powder – 1 Tsp

Cauliflower – 1 Medium head, chopped into florets

Garlic powder - .25 Tsp

Salt – 1.5 Tsp

Juice from 1 lime

Cilantro – 2 Tbsp, chopped

Red Chile Enchilada Chicken:

Red enchilada sauce – 8 Ounce can

Chili powder – 2 Tsp

Chicken breasts – 4 Boneless, skinless

Toppings:

Grilled corn

Black beans

Diced tomatoes

Cilantro

Black olives

In the crock of your slow cooker, cook the red enchilada sauce, chili powder, and chicken for 4-6 hours on a low setting. The meat should be tender and cooked thoroughly.

Once the chicken is cooked, using 2 forks shred the chicken and mix it into the sauce.

Using cold water, rinse the cauliflower, and then dry it using paper towels.

Cut the head of the cauliflower in half using a large, sharp knife and remove the core.

Continue to chop into florets and drop them into a food processor.

Proceed to pulse the cauliflower until it is about the same size as a grain of rice.

(If you do not own a food processor, cauliflower can be riced by hand using a large-hole grater.)

Use cooking spray to spray a large skillet and warm to a medium heat.

Move the riced cauliflower to the skillet and add in the salt, garlic powder, and chili powder.

Saute the cauliflower rice in the pan for about 4 minutes, occasionally stirring.

Stir the chopped cilantro and lime juice in and allow to cook for another minute.

Layer the cauliflower rice first in the bowl, add the shredded chicken, grilled corn, black beans olives, diced tomatoes, and cilantro on top.

Makes 4 servings.

Turkey Taco Bowl

Rice:
Sea salt - .125 Tsp
Uncooked brown rice - .75 Cup
Zest of 1 lime

Turkey:

Lean ground turkey - .75 Pound

Taco seasoning – 2 Tbsp

Salsa:

Cherry tomatoes – 1 Pint, quartered

Jalapeno – 1 Diced

Red onion - .25 Cup, diced

Jalapeno – 1 Diced

Sea salt - .125 Tsp

Juice from ½ of a lime

Cheddar cheese - .25 Cup, shredded

Corn – 1 12 ounce can drained and rinsed

Prepare the brown rice according to the directions on your package, but adding salt and lime zest to the water.

Brown the ground turkey over a mid-level heated cook top burner then mix in your taco seasoning. Allow the turkey to cook until browned. (about 10 minutes)

Mix together all items needed for the salsa until combined well in a small to medium bowl.

Serve by layering cooked rice, corn, turkey meat, and salsa. Top with some shredded cheddar and enjoy.

Makes 4 servings.

Grilled Chicken Wrap with Caesar Salad

Grilled chicken – 8 Ounces, thinly sliced
6 Cups of Kale – 6 Cups cut into small bites
Cherry tomatoes – 1 Cup, quartered
Olive oil - .125 Cup
Parmesan cheese - .5 Cup, finely shredded
Lime juice - .125 Cup, fresh
Coddled egg - .5
Honey – 1 Tsp
Dijon mustard - .5 Tsp
Garlic – 1 Clove, minced
Tortillas – 2 Large
Ground black pepper and sea salt as needed

Whisk together coddled egg, mustard, honey, garlic, olive oil, and lemon juice until well combined to form a dressing. Add pepper and salt as needed.

Add the chicken, kale, tomatoes, and ¼ cup of parmesan to the dressing and mix until well covered.

Layout the tortillas and evenly distribute the salad between them, then sprinkle with ¼ cup of parmesan cheese.

Roll the tortillas into wraps and cut in half to serve.

Makes 2 servings.

Chicken Skillet

Spinach or kale – 3 Cups

Chicken breast or thighs – 1.5 Pounds

Cabbage - .5 Head, chopped

Cilantro - .5 Cup, fresh chopped

Carrots – 3 Grated

Green onions – 6 Chopped

Avocado oil – 3 Tsp

Turmeric – 3 Tsp

Sea salt - .5 Tsp

Powdered garlic – 1 Tsp

Using a large skillet, warm the oil on a burner heated to medium.

Chop the chicken into 1-inch cubes and toss them in with the oil. Fry, the chicken for about 6-8 minutes or until it begins to brown. Stir occasionally.

While the chicken is cooking, chop the cabbage in a food processor.

As the chicken is browning and is just about cooked, add half the cabbage and stir. As the cabbage starts to cook down, add the remaining.

When cabbage has cooked down and softened add in the garlic powder, turmeric, and sea salt. Mix to combine and then incorporate green onions, spinach, and carrots.

Bring the burner heat down to low then stir the mixture until it is well combined.

Allow the chicken mixture to simmer for about 2 to 3 minutes, then take the chicken off of the burner and serve topped with cilantro.

Makes 4 servings.

Lemon Turmeric Chicken

Chicken broth – 1 Cup

Chicken thighs – 4 Bone-in, skin on

Garlic – 3 cloves, minced

Paprika - .5 Tsp

Turmeric – 1 Tsp

1 Lemon

Black pepper - .5 Tsp

Sea salt - .5 Tsp

Paprika - .5 Tsp

Cooking spray or olive oil

Fresh chopped parsley for garnish

Turn oven on to bake at 375 degrees Fahrenheit.

Mix together your spices in a small bowl then season each thigh on both sides and under the skin.

On a medium/high heat, heat a cast-iron skillet. Warm about 2 tbsp of olive oil once the skillet is hot.

Allow the oil time to heat up then lay the chicken skin side down in the skillet. Allow the chicken to cook untouched for roughly 4 minutes before flipping the chicken overtop continue to cook the same on the second side.

Take the chicken out of the skillet and set aside to rest.

Carefully deglaze the skillet by pouring the chicken broth in and scratching at the bottom using a plastic spatula or any non-metal spoon to take up the small pieces that have been stuck. Then squeeze the lemon juice into the broth and add the garlic, then stir well.

Put the meat back into the skillet and cook in the preheated oven for roughly half an hour.

Carefully, take the hot skillet out of the oven, set it aside to let the chicken rest for about 5 minutes.

Serve with greens or wild rice and garnish with the fresh parsley.

Makes 4 servings.

Turmeric Lime Chicken

Chicken breast – 6 Boneless, skinless cutlets
Panko or whole wheat bread crumbs – 2 Cups
Limes - 4Cut in half

Garlic – 3 cloves, minced

Organic eggs - 2 Large, beaten lightly

Cilantro–2 Tbsp

Vegetable oil – 4.5 Tbsp

Turmeric – 1 Tbsp

Pepper and salt as needed

Make 4 small cuts on the top of each chicken breast and season both sides with pepper and salt.

Combine the lime, garlic, and cilantro in a large bowl and let the chicken soak in the marinade covered at room temperature for about 30 minutes.

In one bowl, scramble the eggs. Using a separate bowl, mix together turmeric with the bread crumbs.

Dip each single breast in the egg then lay the chicken in the seasoned bread crumbs to cover.

Over a medium heat, heat about two tablespoons of the vegetable oil in a skillet, then for about 6-10 minutes fry the chicken breasts, flip then continue to cook for an additional 6-10 minutes. Be sure to cook in batches to not crowd the pan with the chicken.

Once chicken is cooked, move it paper towel covered plate to absorb any excess oil.

Enjoy the chicken with steamed vegetables.

Makes 6 servings.

Meatballs

Ground beef – 2 Pounds
Cilantro - .25 Cup, packed
Garlic – 5 Cloves, pressed
Ground ginger - .5 Tsp
Sea salt - .5 Tsp
Zest from 1 lime

Turn oven on to bake at 350 degrees Fahrenheit.

Cover a sheet pan using aluminum foil and put to the side.

Mix together all items using your hands, then shape them into 12 equal-sized balls.

Bake meatballs for 20 to 25 minutes until they are just a little light pink in the middle.

Sprinkle the meatballs with sea salt and serve with a green salad.

Makes 4 servings.

Bacon Cheeseburger Casserole

Ground beef – 2 Pounds

Green onion – 1 Cup, coarsely cut

Sweet potato – 3 Cups, cubed

Coconut cream - .5 of a 13.5 ounce can

Nitrate free bacon – 8 Slices, cooked and crumbled

Sea salt – 1 Tsp

Nutritional yeast - 1 Tsp

Coconut oil – 2 Tbsp

Turn the oven on to bake at 375 degrees Fahrenheit.

Cook the bacon to your liking and let cool.

Steam the sweet potatoes until cooked through but not mushy. You can steam wither using a double boiler or into the microwave with some water until softened.

On a medium heat, melt the coconut oil in a cast-iron skillet. Once the oil has heated, add in the ground beef and ½ teaspoon of sea salt. After cooking for just a few minutes, add in the green onion, and 2-1/2 cups of the steamed potatoes. All to cook until the beef has browned and the sweet potatoes caramelize a little.

Crumble the cooked bacon over the ground beef mixture and stir until well combined.

Shake the can of coconut cream for a minute or so before opening. Pour half of it into a blender and add the yeast, ¼ teaspoon of salt and remaining sweet potato. Blend until well combined.

Pour the sauce from the blender over your ground beef mixture and bake the skillet into the oven for about 5 minutes.

Serve with pickles and red onions.

Makes 6 servings.

Beef and Broccoli

Beef broth – 1 Cup

Boneless chuck roast – 1.5 Pounds sliced into thin strips

Low sodium soy sauce - .5 Cup

Dark brown sugar - .33 Cup

Broccoli florets – 3 Cups, frozen

Garlic – 3 cloves, minced

Cornstarch – 2 Tbsp

Cooked brown rice

Whisk together the brown sugar, sesame oil, broth, soy sauce, and garlic.

Lay the strips of beef in the slow cooker or use a slow cooker liner to allow for easy cleanup.

Pour the broth mix onto the beef and combine until the strips are well covered.

Cook for 5 to 6 hours on low in a covered slow cooker.

Just before the beef is done, remove 4 tablespoons of sauce from the slow cooker and whisk it together with the cornstarch in a small bowl.

Toss the broccoli to the slow cooker and slowly stir the cornstarch mixture in.

Continue to cook until the sauce thickens or for about 30 more minutes.

Serve over the brown rice,

Makes 4-6 servings.

Pot Roast

Chuck roast – 3 Pounds
Water - .75 Cup
Potatoes – 3 Peeled and diced
Carrots – 4 Peeled and sliced
Onion – 1 Quartered
Celery –2 Ribs, sliced
Olive oil – 4.5 Tsp
Worcestershire sauce – 1 Tbsp

Dried basil – 1 Tsp

Beef bouillon granules – 1 Tsp

Ground black pepper and salt as needed

Spray the crock of your slow cooker with non-stick spray, or you can insert a liner.

Into the crock, add the carrots, potatoes, celery, and onion.

Warm the oil in a pot over a mid-level to high burner heat.

Cover all sides of the roast with pepper and salt and brown in the saucepan.

Place the roast on the vegetables in the slow cooker.

Mix the bouillon, Worcestershire, and basil together and pour the mix over the meat and vegetables in the crock.

Cook the roast for 10 hours, covered on low until the beef becomes easy to shred using a fork.

Makes 8 servings.

Almond Butter Beef Stew

Bone broth – 5 Cups

Round steak – 2 Pounds cut to 1.5" cubes

Sweet potatoes – 2 Cups, diced

Carrots – 1 Cup, diced

Onion – 1 Large, finely chopped

Green beans – 1.5 Cups, roughly chopped

Tomatoes – 1.5 Cups, diced

Unsweetened almond butter - .5 Cup

Sea salt – .5 Tbsp

Coconut oil – 3 Tsp

Black pepper - .25 Tsp

Bay leaves - 2

Spray the slow cooker with cooking spray for easy cleaning.

Add all items on the ingredients list, but the green beans to the crock of the slow cooker and mix until well combined.

Cook covered for 6 to 8 hours on low.

When there is just half an hour left to cook, stir in the green beans. Cover again to finish cooking.

Take the bay leaves out and discard. Enjoy it hot.

Makes 5-6 servings.

Liver and Mushroom Stir Fry

Liver – 8 Ounces

Sugar-free, nitrate-free bacon – 8 Ounces

Mushrooms – 8 Ounces

Spinach – 2 or 3 Handfuls

Garlic – 2 Cloves

Slice the liver into thin slices and chop the bacon into small pieces.

Over a medium heat, heat a cast iron pan and cook the bacon pieces. Once done, take the bacon from the pan and transfer it to a paper towel covered plate to allow it to drain. Do not get rid of the bacon grease.

Chop the garlic cloves and cook in the bacon grease until fragrant. Stirring frequently to avoid burning.

Add in the mushrooms and cook them until they just begin to brown. Then drop the spinach into the pan and continue to fry while the spinach begins to wilt, and occasionally stirring. Remove the spinach mushrooms and garlic from the pan, transferring to a bowl but leave the grease.

Place the liver into the cast iron pan carefully to fry it in the grease until it begins to brown, then move all ingredients back to the pan again and stir until well mixed.

Makes 2 servings.

Chicken Hearts with Apples and Carrots

Chicken hearts – 2 Pounds rinsed, cleaned and cut into quarters
White onion – 1 Medium chopped
Apple – 1 Medium, shredded
Carrot – 1 Medium, shredded
Olive oil – 1 Tbsp
Garlic cloves – 2, minced
Black pepper and sea salt as needed
Chopped scallions and parsley for garnish

Warm the oil over a mid-level heated burner on your cook top.

Cook the carrots, garlic, and onion for roughly 3 minutes while occasionally stirring.

Pour the chicken hearts into the skillet and saute for around 10-15 minutes.

Once the chicken has begun to brown, mix into the skillet, the salt, pepper, and apple, then continue to saute for 2 additional minutes.

Move to your serving dish and top with scallions and parsley garnish.

Makes 4 servings.

Moroccan Chicken

Lemon juice – 2 Tbsp

Chicken breast – 1.5 Pounds

Olive oil – 3 Tsp

Powdered cumin – 2 Tsp

Powdered ginger - .5 Tsp

Powdered cinnamon – 1 Tsp

Paprika – 1 Tsp

Turmeric - .5 Tsp

Cayenne - .125 Tsp

Coriander - .125 Tsp

Sea salt - .75 Tsp

Drizzle the chicken with the lemon juice and olive oil in a bowl.

Using another small bowl, stir the salt and spices together and then use it to evenly coat the chicken.

Marinate the chicken in the fridge overnight if possible, no less than 2 hours in a covered bowl.

Add the chicken to a preheated, medium-hot grill. Leave the chicken on the grill until you can see the grill marks, usually about 5 minutes.

Take the chicken off of the direct flames and allow to cook for around 15 to 25 minutes over a low heat. Flip occasionally until the chicken is fully cooked.

Move the chicken overtop a plate and let it sit for about 5 minutes to rest before cutting or serving.

Makes 4 servings.

Lamb kebabs

166

Kebab skewers

Lamb shoulder – 2 Pounds cut into 1" cubes

Garlic – 5 or 6 Cloves

Fresh herbs such as cilantro, parsley, fresh mint, and oregano – 2 Cups

1 Tablespoon of Sea salt – 1 Tbsp

Juice of one lemon

To make the marinade, add all items but the lamb from the list of ingredients into the pitcher of a blender admix until it becomes smooth.

Place the lamb into a bowl and empty the marinade onto it. Use your hands to mix the meat so that it is completely coated. And let sit overnight if possible in the fridge or for at least 1 hour.

If your kebab skewers are wooden, soak in water before use. Slide the lamb onto the skewers and grill them on the BBQ or broil them inside.

Cook the skewers on each side for about 6 to 7 minutes.

Serve the kebabs with cauliflower rice or a green salad.

Makes 6 servings.

Burger and Hot Dog Recipes

<u>Sweet Potato Black Bean Burger</u>

Quinoa - .5 Cup

Sweet potato – 1 Large

Black beans – 1 Can, drained and rinsed

Cilantro- .5 Cup, chopped

Red onion - .5 Cup, diced

Garlic – 2 cloves, minced

Jalapeno - .5, seeded and diced

Spicy Cajun seasoning – 2 Tsp

Cumin – 1 Tsp

Gluten-free oat flour - .25 Cup

Pepper and salt as needed

Olive or coconut oil for cooking

Sprouts

Whole grain hamburger buns - 6

For Avocado-Cilantro Crema:

Low-fat sour cream - .25 Cup

Ripe avocado - .5 Large, diced

Lime juice – 1 Tsp

Cilantro – 2 Tbsp, chopped

Salt as needed

Dash of hot sauce if desired

Use a fine strainer to run water over the quinoa to ensure it is rinsed well.

In medium saucepan, add 8 ounces of water and heat until it reaches a rolling boil.

Once boiling, pour in quinoa and stir while continuing to cook until it returns to boiling.

Once the quinoa has begun to boil, cover, and turn the burner down to low heat. Continue cooking the quinoa until there is no water left in the pan.

Take your saucepan off of the burner on the cook top and use a fork to fluff the quinoa.

Set aside the quinoa in a large bowl for about 10 minutes to allow it to cool.

Poke the sweet potato multiple times using a fork and cook it in the microwave until it is soft and thoroughly cooked about 3 to 4 minutes.

Allow the sweet potato to cool, then remove the skin.

Combine the red onion, beans, cilantro, cooked sweet potato, cumin, Cajun seasoning, and garlic. Pulse in a blending appliance until the mix has little to no lumps. Be sure to incorporate any ingredients stuck to the sides of the bowl while processing the mix.

Add the sweet potato mixture to the quinoa and then add pepper and salt as needed.

Mix the quinoa and sweet potato together and slowly add just enough oat flour to form patties.

Separate the mixture to make 6 patties.

Use parchment paper to cover a baking sheet and place all patties onto the sheet.

Store the patties for at least 30 minutes in the refrigerator to allow the patties to bind together.

In a new bowl or cleaned food processor, place diced avocado, lime juice, sour cream, and cilantro, then mix until combined and all lumps removed.

Add salt if needed, then store the cream in the refrigerator until the burgers are ready to be served.

Over a medium/high heat, warm coconut or olive oil using a large pan.

Pan-fry patties for around 3-4 minutes on each side. Patties are ready when they have browned.

Serve by placing the patties topped with sprouts and avocado cream on whole grain buns.

Makes 6 servings.

Grilled Salmon Burgers

Salmon Burgers:

Salmon fillet – 1 Pound

Almond meal - .5 Cup

Organic egg – 1 Large

Green onions – 2 Chopped

Poblano pepper - .5, seeded and chopped

Salt - .5 Tsp

Fresh lemon juice – 1 Tbsp

Ground black pepper - .25 Tsp

Avocado Salsa:

Green onions, 2 Chopped

Ripe avocado – 1 Large

Poblano pepper - .5, seeded and chopped

Salt - .25 Tsp

Fresh lemon juice – 1 Tbsp

Ground black pepper - .25 Tsp

Using a knife, skin the salmon fillet and chop it into small, bite-sized chunks.

Put the salmon into a large bowl. Add almond meal, egg, poblano, green onion, lemon juice, pepper, and salt, combine well and form 4 patties out of the mixture.

Using another bowl, mix the items needed for the avocado salsa until blended together well.

Cook the salmon burgers on each side for about 3 to 4 minutes over a medium-high heated grill. Be careful not to overcook; you just want the middle of the patty to feel firm.

Top your salmon burgers with the avocado salsa.

Makes 4 servings.

Grilled Carrot "Hot Dogs"

Carrots – 8 Hot dog-sized
Whole-grain hot dog buns– 8
Paprika - .5 Tsp
Liquid smoke – 1.5 Tsp
Powdered garlic - .5 Tsp
Powdered onion - .5 Tsp
Ground mustard - .25 Tsp

Wash and peel the carrots.

Boil the carrots until barely tender, just about 5 to 7 minutes. Do not overcook; you don't want your fork to be able to pierce them.

While the carrots boil, whisk the remaining ingredients to make the marinade.

Take the carrots out of the pot and put them into a storage bag. Add the marinade over the carrots and let sit in the fridge for a minimum of 2 to 3 hours.

Once marinated, the carrots should be grilled for 5 to 7 minutes, until cooked through and grill marks are visible.

Place the carrot dog in a bun and top with your favorite toppings.

Makes 8 servings.

Chicken Zucchini Burger

Chicken breast – 1 Pound
1 Large diced Zucchini – 1 Large, diced
Spring onions – 2 Finely chopped
A large handful of fresh parsley

Garlic – 1 Clove, crushed

Almonds – 3 Tbsp, ground

Paprika – 1 Tsp

Coconut oil – 1 Tbsp

Pepper and salt as needed

Put all items on the ingredients list but the oil into your food processor. Process and combine.

Once the mix becomes smooth and is sticking together, grease your hands and form the mixture into 4 patties.

Warm a non-stick skillet on a mid-level heat and pour in the oil.

Pan-fry the patties 2 at a time on both sides for around 3 or 4 minutes each. Patties are ready once they have become golden brown.

Serve the patties on a green salad or on gluten-free/whole grain buns.

Makes 4 servings.

Lamb and Leek Burgers

Ground lamb – 1 Pound

Leeks - .5 Cup, chopped

Fine sea salt - .5 Tsp

Coconut oil – 1 Tbsp

Garlic powder - .5 Tbsp

Lemon cream:

Coconut cream - .5 Cup

Lemon zest – 1 Tbsp

Using a frying pan, warm 1.5 teaspoons of coconut oil on a mid-level heat and cook the leeks for about 3 to 5 minutes until they have softened.

Move the leeks to a bowl and give them some time to cool.

Add the lamb, oil, garlic, salt, and cooled leeks to a large bowl and then use your hands to mix them until well combined.

Make 4 patties out of the lamb mixture.

Add the remaining coconut oil to the frying pan, then cook all patties over a mid-level heated burner for about 5 minutes per side until the patties are browned.

In a small blender, mix the zest and the cream.

Top the patties with the lemon cream and serve the patties with a wild rice or greens, or on a gluten-free bun.

Makes 4 servings.

Herb burgers

Ground beef or bison – 1 Pound

Dried thyme - .75 Tsp

Dried sage - .5 Tsp

Sea salt - .5 Tsp

Dried rosemary - .25 Tsp

Use your hands to mix together all of the items in the list of ingredients in a large bowl. Mix well.

Make 4 evenly sized patties out of the mixture and let them sit for about 30 minutes.

Cook on each side for around 3 to 5 minutes over a mid-level heated burner using a nonstick frying pan.

Serve with greens of on a whole wheat/gluten-free bun.

Makes 4 servings.

Cinnamon Sliders

Ground beef – 2 Pounds
Cinnamon – 2 Tsp
Sea salt – 1 Tsp

In a large bowl, mix all items together using just your hands.

Once they are blended well, shape mixture into 8 patties and cook over a medium/high heat on your cook top for about 6 to 11 minutes. Turn the patties over and continue to cook until browned on both sides.

Would be great cooked on a BBQ grill too!

Makes 8 servings.

<u>Veggie Burgers</u>

Black beans – 3 Cups, rinsed, drained and cooked

Cashews – 1 Cup

Water - .5 Cup

Brown rice – 1.5 Cups, cooked

Parsley - .5 Cup, chopped

Carrots – 1.5 Cups, shredded

Gluten-free bread crumbs – 1 Cup

Ground flax - .25 Cup

Green onions - .33 Cup

Mix the flax and water until combined then put to the side until needed.

Mash the black beans using a fork in a large bowl until they form a paste but still leaving about ¼ of the beans whole.

Put the cashews in a food processor until they have been broken down to a large bread crumb size. Add the cashews, flax mix, and all remaining ingredients to the large bowl of black beans and stir together until the mixture has been combined well using a wooden spoon.

Use about ½ cup of the mixture to form each patty about ¾" thick.

Over a medium heat, heat about 2 to 3 tbsp of oil.

Cook the patties in batches of 4 for 3 to 4 minutes per side until they become crispy and golden.

Move the patties to a plate covered with paper towels. Allow them to draw off any excess grease.

Serve each patty on a gluten-free bun with your favorite toppings.

Makes 12 servings.

Chicken Burgers

Mint leaves – 1 Cup, loosely packed
Ground chicken – 1 Pound
Yellow onion – 1 Medium, finely diced
Coconut flour – 2 Tbsp
Zested lemon – 1 Tbsp
Ground ginger – 2 Tsp
Turmeric – 1 Tsp

Salt – .75 Tsp

Lemon juice – 1 Tbsp

Turn the oven on to bake at 390 degrees Fahrenheit.

Add the ginger, ground chicken, lemon juice and zest, mint leaves, turmeric, and salt and process them together in a food processor until they are combined well.

Process again after adding flour to the mixture.

Make 18 small burgers out of the mixture and bake for about 20 minutes on a greased baking pan.

Makes 18 burgers.

Fish Burgers

Sardines – 1 3.75 ounce can drained

Wild salmon – 1 14.75 ounce can drained

Organic egg – 1 Large

Coconut oil – 2.25 Tbsp

Flaxseed meal – 2 Tbsp, ground

Dijon mustard – 1.25 Tsp

Red onion – 2 Tbsp, diced

Paprika - .5 Tsp

Fresh dill – 2 Tbsp, chopped

Sea salt - .5 Tsp

Turmeric - .25 Tsp

Ground black pepper

First, be sure to drain the salmon and sardines well then remove any large pieces of skin and bone from the salmon.

Add the fish and all remaining items on the list of ingredients, except for the oil into a blender or a food processor. Mix the ingredients together.

Once smooth and well combined, warm3 tsp of coconut oil in a large frying pan over a mid-level to high heat burner.

Drop large tbsp's of the fish mixture into the heated frying pan before flattening slightly using your spatula.

Cover the frying pan and bring the burner down to a mid-level heat. Allow to continue frying for around 3 to 4 minutes. Remove the cover and flip the patties, patting them down again, and cook the remaining side for another 2 to 3 minutes. Move them to a plate covered in paper towels covered plate and repeat for the remaining fish mixture.

Makes 10-11 burgers.

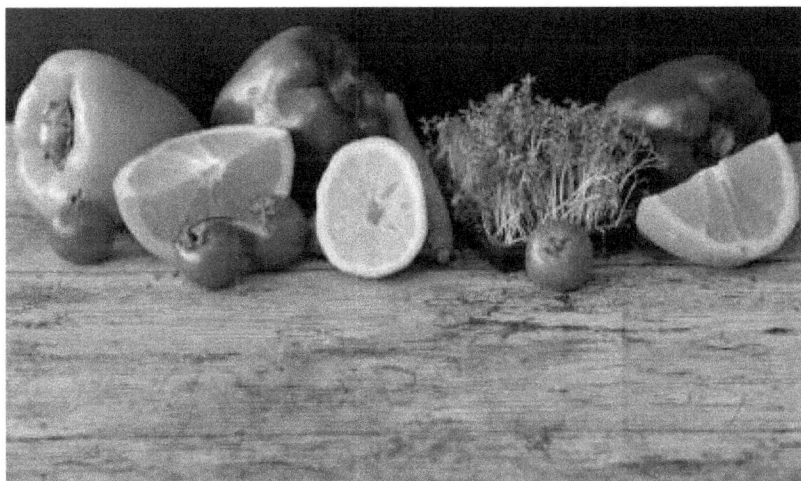

Condiments, Sauces, and Dressings

Turmeric Tahini Dressing

Water - .33 Cup

Tahini - .25 Cup

Garlic – 1 Small clove, finely minced

Apple cider vinegar – 3 Tsp

Tamari – 3 Tsp

Lemon juice – 3 Tsp, freshly squeezed

Turmeric – .75 Tsp

Maple syrup - .5 Tsp

Ginger – 1 Tsp, finely grated

Whisk all ingredients together until they are mixed well.

Store in the refrigerator in a well-sealed glass jar for no longer than 5 days.

Carrot Ketchup

Carrot – 12 Ounces

Beets – 6 Ounces, chopped

Honey – .125 Cup

No sugar added apple juice - .25 Cup

Apple cider vinegar – 1.75 Tbsp

Sea salt -.5 Tsp

Powdered onion - .5 Tsp

Powdered ginger - .25 Tsp

Powdered garlic - .25 Tsp

Insert a steaming basket over a large pot and add water to just about an inch below the steamer.

Put the beets and carrots in the basket and heat water to boiling. Once boiling, turn down the burner to low/midlevel and allow to cook for 12-15 additional minutes covered.

Once the vegetables are soft, remove them from the steamer and combine them in a blender with the remaining items on the list of the ingredients. Pulse and mix   until you get a smooth sauce.

Pour the "ketchup" into a small saucepan, cook on a low simmer for 18-20 minutes at medium-low heat.

"Ketchup" may be kept in a well-sealed glass jar no longer than 3 days in the refrigerator. Or store in the freezer and thaw out as needed.

Garlic Artichoke Spread

Artichoke hearts – 2 Cups
Coconut oil - .125 Cup
Garlic – 4 cloves, minced
Lemon juice - .5 Tbsp, freshly squeezed
Sea salt - .25 Tsp
Dried oregano - .5 Tbsp

Turn the oven on to bake at 400 degrees Fahrenheit.

Mix all items in the ingredients listand arrange into a small glass baking pan.

Place a sheet of aluminum foil over the top and cook the spread in the oven for 45 to 50 minutes and stir once, about halfway through.

 Take the spread out of the oven and allow to cool. Then pour the spread into your food processor and pulse together for a chunky spread.

Makes 4 servings.

Guacamole

Avocados - 5
White wine vinegar – 1 Tbsp
Fine sea salt – 1 Tsp
Juiced lemon - 1
Powdered onion - 1.5 Tsp
Powdered Garlic – 1.5 Tsp

Discard the stone from the avocados and cut into quarters.

Scoop the avocado meat into a blender and add garlic, vinegar, onion, lemon juice, and sea salt.

Pulse until well blended, scraping down the side to ensure all ingredients are mixed together.

Taste the mixture and adjust seasoning accordingly.

Once thoroughly combined, scrape the guacamole into an airtight storage container.

May be kept in the fridge in a sealed jar for up to 7 days, or you can freeze it in a freezer-safe container for months.

Makes 5-6 cups.

Nightshade Free Salsa

Beets - .33 Cup of drained and rinsed
Carrots – 1 14.5 ounce can drained and rinsed
White onion – 1 Small
Sea salt - .5 Tsp
Lime juiced – 2 or 3 Tbsp, fresh squeezed
Cilantro - .5 Bunch, rinsed

Pulse all items on the list of ingredients in a blender until well blended but still somewhat chunky.

Serve chilled.

Makes 2 cups.

Turmeric Sauerkraut

Cabbage – 1 Medium head
Turmeric – 2.5 Tsp
Garlic – 1 Large clove, grated

Fine sea salt – .5 Tbsp

Jalapeno - .5, diced small

Wash the cabbage and tear a large leaf off of the outside layer then set aside.

Grate the cabbage into a large bowl or shred using a mandolin.

Using gloves, massage the cabbage and mix in all of the other ingredients while slightly squeezing the cabbage to release the juices.

After a few minutes of massaging the ingredients in the bowl, the cabbage should have shrunk down to about half the volume.

Put the sauerkraut and liquid into a glass jar and pack tightly. Pack until the cabbage mix leaves about an inch of space between the mix and the jar top. Push the sauerkraut down further to allow the liquid to rise above the cabbage.

Place the large cabbage leaf that you had set aside, on top of the jar to keep the sauerkraut below the liquid. Cut down leaf if needed.

Seal the jar tightly and leave it out in a sunny area of your countertop.

Each day open lid to release any pressure and reclose.

Leave on counter for a week or two to allow it to ferment until it reaches the desired taste.

The sauerkraut should be bubbly and sour tasting.

Makes 8 servings.

Turmeric Dressing

Lemon juice – .125 Cup
Extra virgin olive oil - .25 Cup
Ground turmeric – 1 Tsp
Raw honey – 2 Tsp
Avocado - .5
Sea salt - .25 Tsp

Combine all ingredients together in a blender. The avocado will make it a thicker dressing or dip. Add in until it reaches your desired consistency.

Raspberry Vinaigrette

Olive oil - .75 Cup
Water - .25 Cup
Apple cider vinegar -.25 Cup
Dried basil – 1 Tsp
Raspberries - .5 Cup (fresh or frozen)
Fine sea salt – 1 Tsp

Combine all items from the list of ingredients in a blender and mix together until they reach a smooth consistency.

Avocado Dill Sauce

Avocado - 1
Juiced lemon - .5
1Garlic – 1 Clove
A bunch of dill

Peel the avocado and remove the pit. Chop the dill, press the garlic and add all items on the list of ingredients to a blender.

Process in blender until the sauce becomes smooth.

Golden Hummus

Chickpeas – 1 15 ounce can drained
Juiced lemon – 1 Medium
Ginger – .5 Tbsp, grated
Olive oil – 1.5 Tbsp
Tahini – 3 Tbsp
Turmeric - .5 Tsp, grated
Turmeric - .25 Tsp, ground
Garlic – 2 cloves, minced
Fine sea salt - .25 Tsp
A pinch of cayenne

Mix all items on the ingredients list together in a blender and combine together until it becomes smooth.

Taste the hummus and adjust seasoning as needed.

Store for 3 to 4 days in the refrigerator using an airtight container.

Coconut Milk Ranch Dressing

Coconut cream – 1 Can (ingredients should be just coconut and water)

Shallots – 2 Tbsp, minced

Chives – .125 Cup, chopped

Apple cider vinegar – 2.25 Tbsp

Basil – 1.5 Tbsp, chopped

Dill – 2.75 Tsp, chopped

Parsley–2 Tbsp, chopped

Fine sea salt – .75 Tsp

Garlic – 1 Clove, minced

Open the coconut cream and scoop out the cream leaving the water in the can.

Whisk together the cream with the 4 Tablespoons of the coconut water.

Once well combined, mix the remaining items on the list of ingredients into the bowl and blend together until they are well blended.

Before serving, allow the flavors to combine by storing in the fridge for at least 30 minutes.

Mustard

Apple cider vinegar - .25 Cup

Raw honey – 1 Tbsp

Ground mustard - .5 Cup

Fine sea salt - .25 Tsp

Ground turmeric - .25 Tsp

Stir all ingredients until well combined in a small mixing bowl.

May be kept in a well-sealed jar in the fridge.

Hot Sauce

Apple cider vinegar - .25 Cup

Tomato paste – 1 Tbsp

Water - .25 Cup

Paprika - .25 Tsp

Cayenne - .5 Tsp

Fine sea salt - .25 Tsp

Flaked red pepper - .125 Tsp

Powdered garlic - .125 Tsp

Using a mixing bowl, stir all items on the list of ingredients together until combined well.

May be kept in a well-sealed jar in the fridge.

Mayonnaise

Organic egg – 1 Large
Avocado oil – 8 Ounces
Apple cider vinegar – 1.5 Tbsp
Dijon mustard – 1.25 Tsp
Fine sea salt - .25 Tsp

Combine vinegar, mustard egg and sea salt in a blender.

Slowly drizzle the avocado oil through the funnel while the blender is running and continue to blend until it thickens.

Once avocado oil is well combined, pour the mayo into an airtight jar and store in the refrigerator.

Dandelion Pesto

Dandelion leaves – 2 Cups, chopped and loosely packed

Pine nuts - .5 Cup

Parmesan cheese - .25 Cup, freshly grated

Olive oil–4 Ounces

Garlic Cloves - 3Minced

Lemon juice – 1 Tbsp

Sea salt - .5 Tsp

Lemon zest – 1 Tbsp

Turmeric powder -1 Tsp

Add all items from the list of ingredients, less the cheese into a blender and combine until they become smooth.

Add a small amount of olive oil if the pesto is too thick until it reaches your desired consistency.

Mix in the parmesan and blend once again until combined and smooth.

May be kept in an airtight container in the fridge for no longer than 72 hours.

Smoothies and Drinks

Green Smoothie

Banana – 1 Frozen and sliced

Fresh kale – .75 Cup

Unsweetened nut milk – 8 Ounces

Turmeric - .25", Peeled and sliced

Fresh ginger - .25", peeled and sliced

Chia seeds - .5 Tsp

Ground cinnamon - .25 Tsp

Flax seeds - .5 Tsp

Add all items together in your blending appliance and mix. Once well incorporated and liquified, pour into your glass and enjoy.

Cherry Banana Smoothie

Organic cherries – 1 Cup

Ripe bananas - 2

Baby spinach– 1 Cup

Coconut water – .75 Cup

Ginger – 1 Tsp, freshly grated

Powdered turmeric - .5 Tsp

Pre-soaked chia seeds – .75 Tsp

Powdered Cinnamon - .25 Tsp

Using a blender, blend together all ingredients until smooth.

Cherry Mango Smoothie

Sweet cherries – 1 Cup, frozen

Mango – 1 Cup, frozen

Water - .5 Cup

Water - .75 Cup

First, place the cherries and the mangoes into separate bowls and leave them out to thaw.

Mix the cherries and 4 ounces of water in your blending appliance and blend together.

You may add an extra ¼ cup of the water if you would like to thin it out some then pour it into a glass.

Rinse out the blender and add the mango and the remaining water. Blend until smooth, adding additional water if needed.

Pour into glass over the cherry layer.

Blueberry Smoothie

Almond milk – 1 Cup
Banana – 1 Frozen
Blueberries – 1 Cup, frozen
Spinach – 2 Handfuls
Cinnamon - .25 Tsp
Almond butter – 1 Tbsp
Cayenne - .125 Tsp

Place the items into your blending appliance then process. Once smooth, pour into your cups and enjoy.

Golden Milk

Light coconut milk – 1.5 Cups
Unsweetened, nut milk – 1.5 Cups
Powdered ginger - .25 Tsp
Powdered turmeric – .5 Tbsp
Powdered cinnamon - .25 Tsp

Coconut oil – 1 Tbsp

Your choice of sweetener such as coconut sugar, maple syrup, etc.

Whisk the items together using a small pot then warm on a mid-level heated cook top.

Continue to whisk frequently until milk is hot to the touch but not boiling.

Turn off the heat and taste to adjust ingredients as necessary.

Remove the cinnamon stick and serve immediately.

Makes 2 servings.

Turmeric Hot Chocolate

Unsweetened almond milk – 1 Cup

Unsweetened cocoa powder – 1.5 Tbsp

Coconut oil – 2 Tsp

Honey – 2 Tsp

Ground turmeric – 1 Tsp

A pinch of cayenne pepper

A pinch of ground black pepper

Pour the milk into a saucepan and add the cocoa, coconut oil, and turmeric. Whisk together and bring to a boil.

Take the pan off of the stovetop then add in the pepper and cayenne.

Let sit for 2 minutes before serving.

Beet and Cherry Smoothie

Beets – 2 Small, ready to eat, cut into quarters

Unsweetened vanilla almond milk – 10 Ounces

Banana - .5 Frozen

Pitted cherries - .5 Cup, frozen

Almonds – 1 Tbsp

Mix all items together in your blending appliance. Ready to serve once well mixed and liquified.

Pineapple Smoothie

Chunks of Pineapple – 1.5 Cup, from freezer

Coconut water – 1.25 Cup

Orange – 1 Peeled

Fresh ginger – 1 Tbsp, finely chopped

Ground turmeric – 1.25 Tsp

Black pepper - .25 Tsp

Chia seeds – .75 Tsp

Mix all items in your blending appliance.

Ready to serve once smooth.

Greek Yogurt Smoothie

Unsweetened almond milk – 1 Cup

Baby spinach - .25 Cu

Plain Greek yogurt - .5 Cup

Blueberries - .25 Cup, fresh or frozen

Almond butter – 1 Tbsp

Ice cubes – 3 or 4

Mix the items together in a blending appliance.

Ready to serve once smooth.

Cacao Smoothie

Coconut milk – 1 cup
Cacao powder – 3 Tbsp
Raspberries – 1.25 Cup, frozen
Filtered water - .5 Cup
Banana - 1
Honey – 1 Tbsp
Baby spinach – .75 Cup

Combine the items in a blending appliance. Once it has liquified and is well mixed, pour into cups.

Serve immediately.

Golden Milk Latte

Almond milk – 2 or 3 Cups
Vanilla extract - .25 Tsp
Maple syrup – 3 Tbsp
Powdered cinnamon - .25 Tsp
Powdered turmeric – .66 Tbsp

Powdered ginger - .25 Tsp

A pinch of ground black pepper

A pinch of ground cardamom

Combine the items in a cocktail or shaker bottle.

Shake until well combined and pour over ice.

Use 2 cups of milk for a sweeter spiced drink or 3 cups for a milder drink.

Golden Milkshake

Unsweetened almond milk – 2 Cups

Almond butter – 2 Tbsp

Raw honey – .125 Cup

Coconut oil – 3 Tsp

Powdered cinnamon – .33 Tbsp

Powdered turmeric – 1.5 Tbsp

Powdered ginger - .5 Tsp

A pinch of black pepper

Add all items to a blending appliance starting with just 1/3 of the honey and adding more if you desire a sweeter milkshake.

Blend until smooth and serve immediately.

For a thicker milkshake, freeze the milk in ice cube trays before blending.

Carrot and Ginger Smoothie

Carrots – 3 Cups,.5 grated
Plain yogurt - .25 Cup
Coconut milk – 1 cup
Grated ginger - 1
A handful of ice
Honey - Tbsp

In a blender, mix together all ingredients until they become smooth.

Tart Cherry Smoothie

Tart cherries - 1 Cup, frozen
Water – 8 Ounces, filtered
Ice - .5 Cup

Tart cherry juice, 4 Ounces

Apple – 1Cut in half, core removed

Peeled orange - 1

Banana – 1 Frozen

Blend all ingredients together until completely smooth.

Power Smoothie

Vanilla Greek yogurt - .5 Cup

Orange juice – 1 Cup, freshly squeezed

Whole grain oats - .25 Cup

Baby spinach - 3 Cups

Blueberries – 1.5 Cups, frozen

Ice – 1 Cup

Banana - 1

Combine all ingredients together until smooth in a blender.

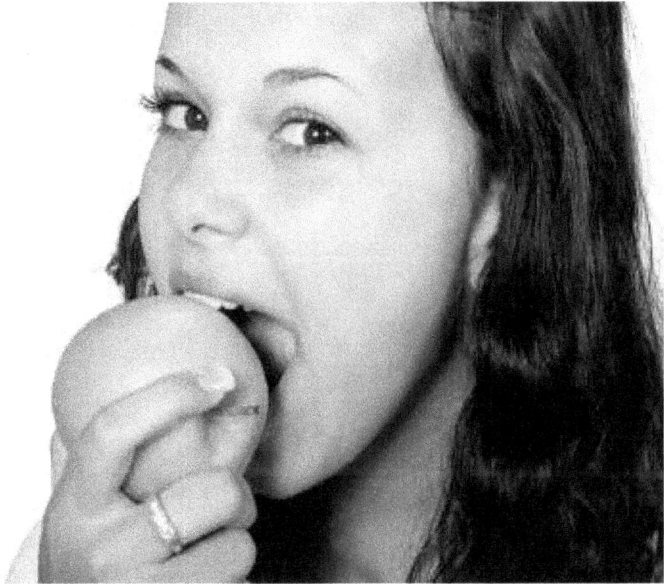

Desserts and Snacks

<u>Chocolate Dipped Bananas</u>

Dark chocolate – 12 Ounces

Bananas – 1 Large cut into thirds

Coconut oil – 1 Tbsp

Chopped, salted pistachios

Chopped, smoked almonds

Cocoa nibs

Popsicle sticks

In a double boiler, melt together the chocolate and coconut oil, stirring until smooth.

Use a silicone pad to cover a cookie pan and put to the side until needed.

Into one end of each banana, insert a Popsicle stick and dip the bananas into the chocolate, lightly tapping them on the side of the pot to remove excess.

Lay the bananas out onto the parchment and sprinkle with the chopped nuts and cocoa nibs.

Place in the baking sheet in the freezer to allow the bananas to harden and set.

Once fully frozen, serve or wrap individually to store in the freezer.

Makes 9 servings.

Cinnamon Apple Chips

Fuji apples – 3 large

Ground cinnamon- .75 Tsp

Place your oven racks in the upper and lower portions of the oven and set to 200 degrees Fahrenheit.

Cover 2 cookie sheets with silicone pads then put to the side until needed.

Wash the apples then remove the cores using an apple corer.

Using a mandolin, slice the apples to 1/8" thick slices.

Lay the apples out over the baking sheets and an even, single layer.

Sprinkle the apples with cinnamon and bake each pan on an upper and lower rack for 60 minutes.

After the 1 hour, take the pans and switch racks to move the pan that was on the upper rack to the lower and the one that was on the lower rack to the upper.

Continue to bake for 1-1/2 hours.

Test the doneness by removing 1 chip from a pan and letting it cool outside the oven for 2-3 minutes. If it is crispy after cooling, it is done.

Turn the oven off but let the apples stay in there for another hour to allow to cool and crisp.

Makes about 6 servings.

Avocado Brownies

Ripe avocado – 1 Large
Organic eggs – 3 Large
Unsweetened apple sauce - .5 Cup
Sea salt - .25 Tsp
Coconut flour - .5 Cup
Maple syrup - .5 Cup
Baking soda – 1 Tsp
Unsweetened Dutch cocoa powder - .5 Cup
Vanilla extract – .33 Tbsp

Turn on the stove to bake at 350 degrees Fahrenheit.

In your blender, combine the vanilla, maple syrup, avocado, and apple sauce.

Move the ingredients to a large bowl, add eggs, and whisk together.

Stir in the coconut flour, sea salt, cocoa, and baking soda. Continue stirring until well combined.

Use coconut oil to grease an 8x8 baking pan and pour in the batter.

Allow to bake in oven for about 25 minutes.

Once the brownies have cooled for 20 minutes, cut into 16 pieces.

Store the brownies unrefrigerated in an airtight container for up to 2 days.

Makes 16 servings.

Frozen Blueberry Bites

Vanilla yogurt – 8 Ounces

Lemon juice – 2 Tsp

Blueberries - Pint, fresh

Using your hands or a wooden spoon, gently mix the ingredients together in a large bowl so that blueberries are not squished.

Cover a cookie sheet with a silicone pad and scoop the yogurt covered blueberries out onto it.

Store the baking sheet in the freezer for about 2 hours before serving.

Spice Cookies

Palm shortening or butter – 8 Tbsp

Cassava flour – 1.5 Cups

Coconut sugar - .66 Cups

Organic eggs, 3 Large

Ground turmeric – 1 Tbsp

Organic blackstrap molasses – 3 Tsp

Ground ginger – 2.75 Tsp

Ground black pepper–3 Tsp

Cinnamon – .75 Tbsp

Salt - .25 Tbsp

Orange extract- .25 Tbsp

Baking soda – .25 Tbsp

Set the stove to bake at 350 degrees Fahrenheit.

Use silicone baking pads to cover 2 cookie sheets.

Use a hand mixer to mix together sugar, shortening, eggs, and molasses until well combined.

Add in the orange extract, salt, spices, and baking soda and continue mixing.

Slowly pour in the cassava and continue with the hand mixer until it forms a dough.

Lay a sheet of parchment or wax paper out flat on your countertop and smooth and thin out your dough using a rolling pin until the thickness is about ¼"-3/8".

Use a cookie cutter to cut out cookies and lay them out on the cookie sheets.

Bake until the cookies are slightly golden, about 13-15 minutes.

Move the cookies to allow to cool on a cooling rack.

Makes about 18 cookies.

Pumpkin Spice Cookies

Pumpkin puree – 1.5 Cups

Unsweetened coconut flakes – 1 Cup

Maple syrup - .5 Cup

Coconut flour - .33 Cup

Ground cinnamon – 1.5 Tsp

Coconut oil - .33 Cup

Ginger - .75 Tsp

Turn on the stove to bake at 350 degrees Fahrenheit.

Line a cookie pan with a piece of parchment paper

Use a mixer to combine all items in the recipe until they form a batter.

Using a tablespoon or cookie scoop, scoop out even sized cookies and arrange on the parchment paper, then flatten them slightly.

After 30 minutes of baking time, remove the cookies, and set them on a cooling rack.

Store the cookies at room temperature uncovered for a hard cookie or covered it. You prefer a softer cookie.

Banana Coconut Cookies

Banana - 1
Unsweetened, shredded coconut - .75 Cup

Set the oven to 350 degrees Fahrenheit.

Use coconut oil or spray to grease a cookie sheet and set aside.

Use a blender to pulse all items on the list of ingredients.

Once combined, shape the batter into disks and arrange onto a cookie sheet.

Put the sheet into the preheated oven for about 25 minutes until they are just beginning to brown. Transfer to a cooling rack.

Ginger Date Bars

Dates - .75 Cup
Almond flour – 1 Cup
Ground ginger – 1 Tsp
Unsweetened almond milk - .25 Cup

Set oven to 350 degrees Fahrenheit.

Add dates and almond milk to the blender and mix until the ingredients combine into a paste.

Add the almond flour and ginger to the paste and continue to blend for 2-3 minutes.

Bake the mixture for 20 minutes in an 8x8 baking dish.

Allow to cool, then slice into 8 bars.

Makes 8 servings.

Spicy Nuts

Almonds – 1 Cup

Olive oil – 1 Tbsp

Cashews – 1.25 Cup

Cayenne pepper – 1 Tsp

Paprika-.25 Tsp

Pecans – .75 Cup

Cumin - .75 Tsp

Garlic powder - .75 Tsp

Ground black pepper - .5 Tsp

½ Teaspoon of Sea salt - .5 Tsp

Set stove to bake at 350 degrees Fahrenheit.

Cover a sheet pan with foil, then arrange the nuts on the pan, so none are overlapping.

Cook the nuts for7 minutes, turn and continue to roast for an additional 7 to 8 minutes.

While the nuts are roasting, stir the chili powder, cumin, garlic, salt, black pepper, and cayenne until well combined in a small bowl.

Take the nuts out of the oven and put them to the side to cool. Transfer the nuts to a large bowl and coat with oil, then the spice mix. Stir until well coated.

Store in a sealed container at room temperature.

Lemon Garlic Plantain Chips

Green plantains sliced into chips – 3 Cups
Avocado oil – 3 Tbsp
Garlic powder – 2 Tsp
Lemon juice – 1 Tbsp

Set the stove to bake at 350 Degrees Fahrenheit.

Lightly grease or cover a sheet pan with parchment paper and set aside.

Using a slightly larger mixing bowl, add the plantain slices and gently coat with the coconut oil and garlic using your hands.

Once the oven is heated, coat the plantains with the lemon juice and toss again to make sure they are fully coated.

Arrange the plantains across the baking sheet so that they do not overlap and bake until they just begin to brown.

Remove the plantains and move them to a plate covered with paper towels to drain and cool before serving.

Chocolate Chiai Pudding

Unsweetened almond milk – 2 Cups
Maple syrup - .25 Cup plus 2 tbsp
Cocoa powder - .25 Cup
Chia seeds - .25 Cup plus 2 tbsp
A pinch of sea salt

Using a whisk, mix all ingredients in an average-sized mixing bowl. Continue to mix until the cocoa powder has fully dissolved, and the pudding is combined well.

Place the bowl in the refrigerator, covered for about 6 hours while occasionally stirring to allow time for the chia seeds to turn jelly-like and the pudding can set.

Makes 4 servings.

Watermelon Sorbet

1 Seedless watermelon – 1Peeled and cubed

Place a single layer of watermelon cubes in a baking pan and freeze for about 2 hours until the watermelon is solid.

Put the watermelon into a food processor and mix. Once the watermelon has reached a soft, slightly thick consistency, transfer it to a deep baking dish making sure to pack it in tight.

Put the pan in the freezer for about 1-2 hours until the sorbet is scoop able.

Sunshine Smoothie Bowl

Bananas – 1 or 2, Frozen
Pineapple - .5 Cup, frozen
Coconut cream– 2 or 3 Tsp
Mango - .5 Cup, frozen
Elderflower syrup – 2 Tsp
Coconut milk - .25 Cup
Lucuma – 1 Tsp

Add all items in the ingredient list and mix in a blending appliance. Once the smoothie is well mixed and liquified, transfer the smoothie to a bowl, then cover with toasted coconut or dried pineapple if desired.

Tropical Smoothie Bowl

Smoothie:
Mango – 16 ounces, from freezer
Banana - .5
Pineapple – 16 ounces, from freezer
Chia seeds – 2.5 Tsp
Orange juice – 1 Cup
Turmeric - .125 Tsp

Toppings:
Chopped almonds
Coconut flakes
Sliced kiwi
Sliced strawberry

Combine all items listed in the smoothie ingredients and mixing a blender. Once the ingredients have been well broken down and thoroughly mixed, transfer the smoothie to a bowl and cover with strawberries, kiwi, nuts, and coconut.

Turmeric Mango Smoothie Bowl

Smoothie:

Banana – 1 Frozen

Mangos - .5 Cup, frozen

Plain, unsweetened yogurt - .5 Cup

Dates -2

Almond butter, 2 Tbsp

Ground turmeric - .5 Tsp

Flaxseed meal – 2 Tbsp

A splash of unsweetened almond milk

A pinch of salt

Toppings:

Granola

Coconut Flakes

Blend all smoothie ingredients together until smooth.

Pour the smoothie into a bowl and sprinkle with granola and coconut.

Conclusion

Thank you for making it through to the end of *The Anti-Inflammatory Diet for Beginners*, let's hope it was enjoyable and informative and has provided you with aloof the tools you need to achieve your goals whatever they may be.

The next step is to put this new information to action. Go to the grocery store and fill that cart with colorful, anti-inflammatory foods and start your new healthy, pain-free life .

Finally, if you found this book has changed your life or is useful in anyway, a review on Amazon is always appreciated!

www.ingramcontent.com/pod-product-compliance
Lightning Source LLC
Chambersburg PA
CBHW060317030426
42336CB00011B/1095